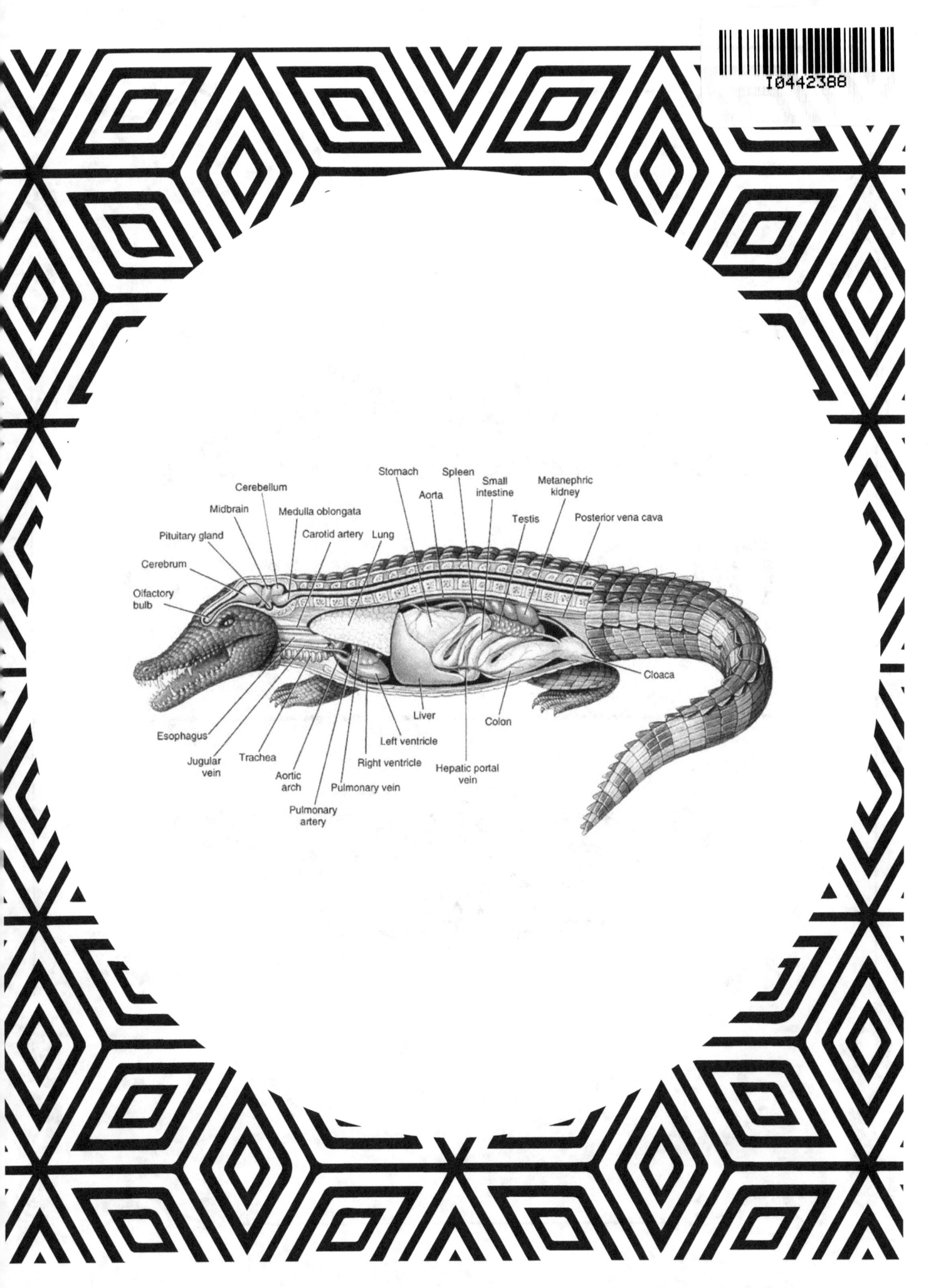

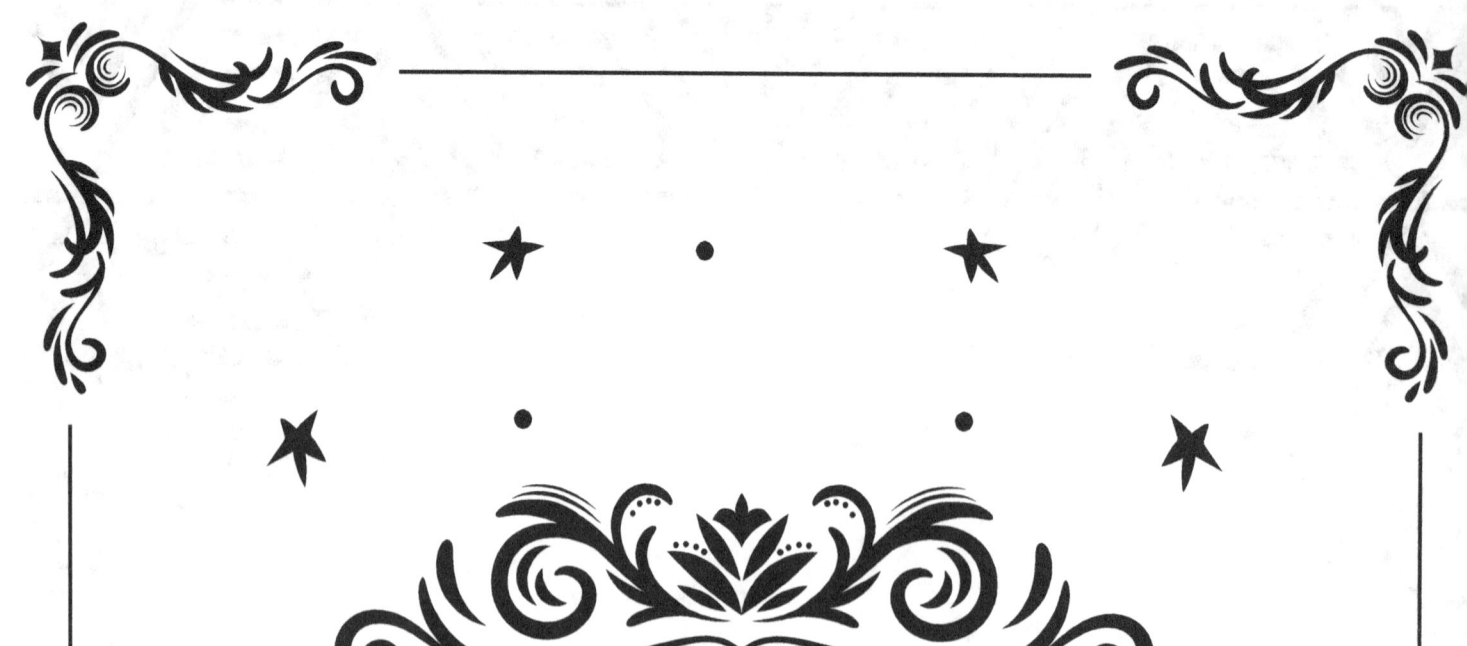

This Book Belongs To

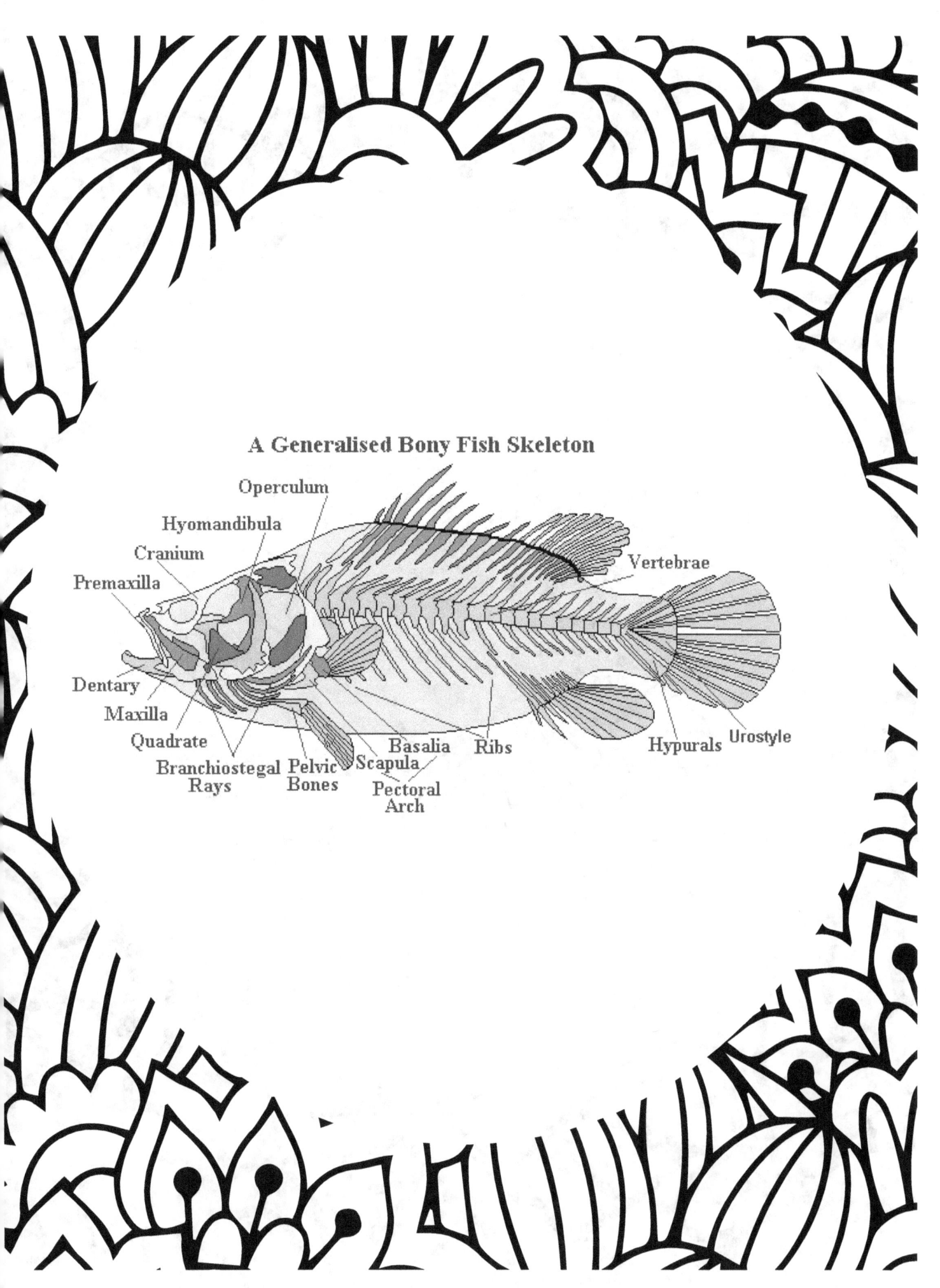

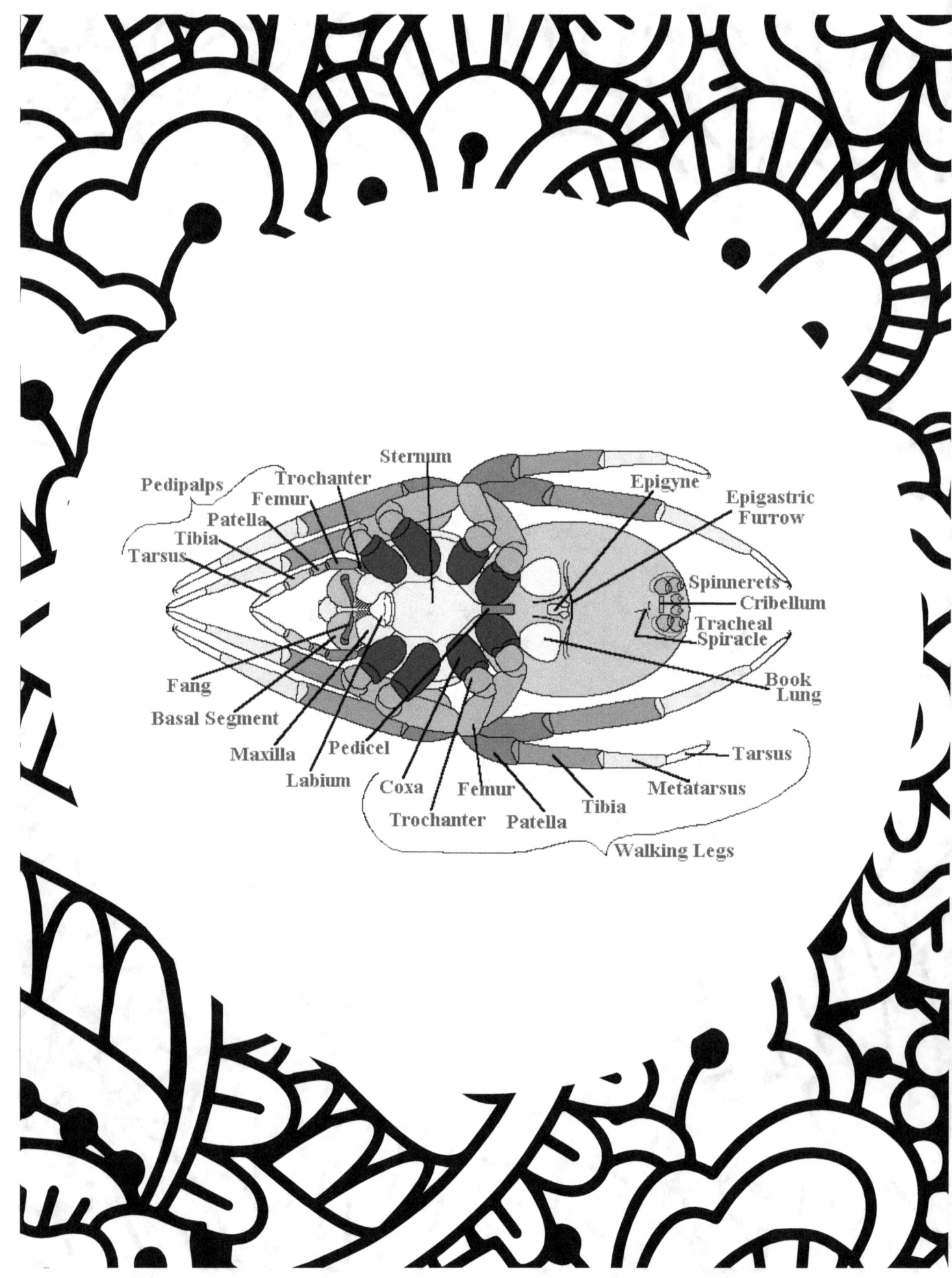

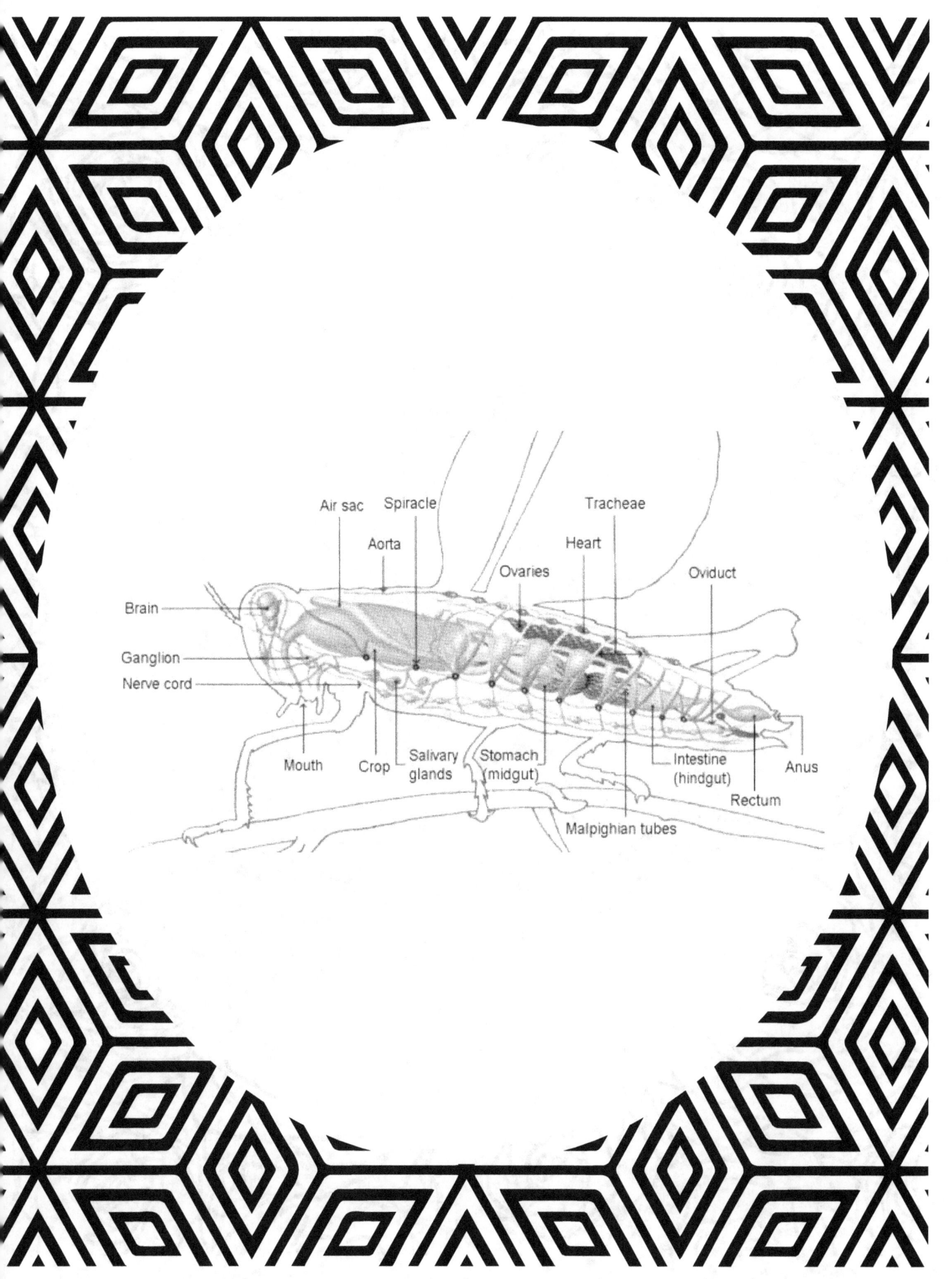

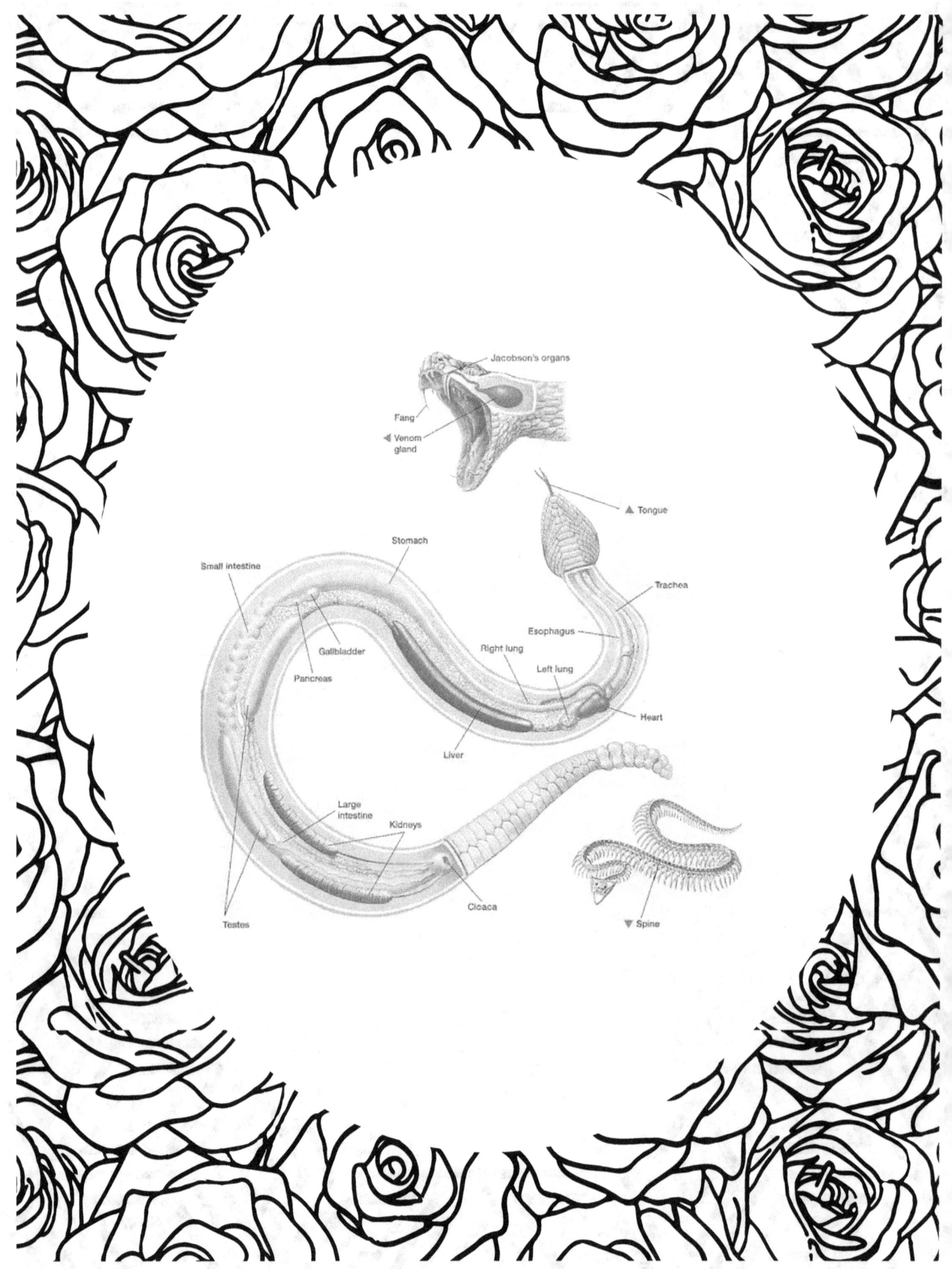

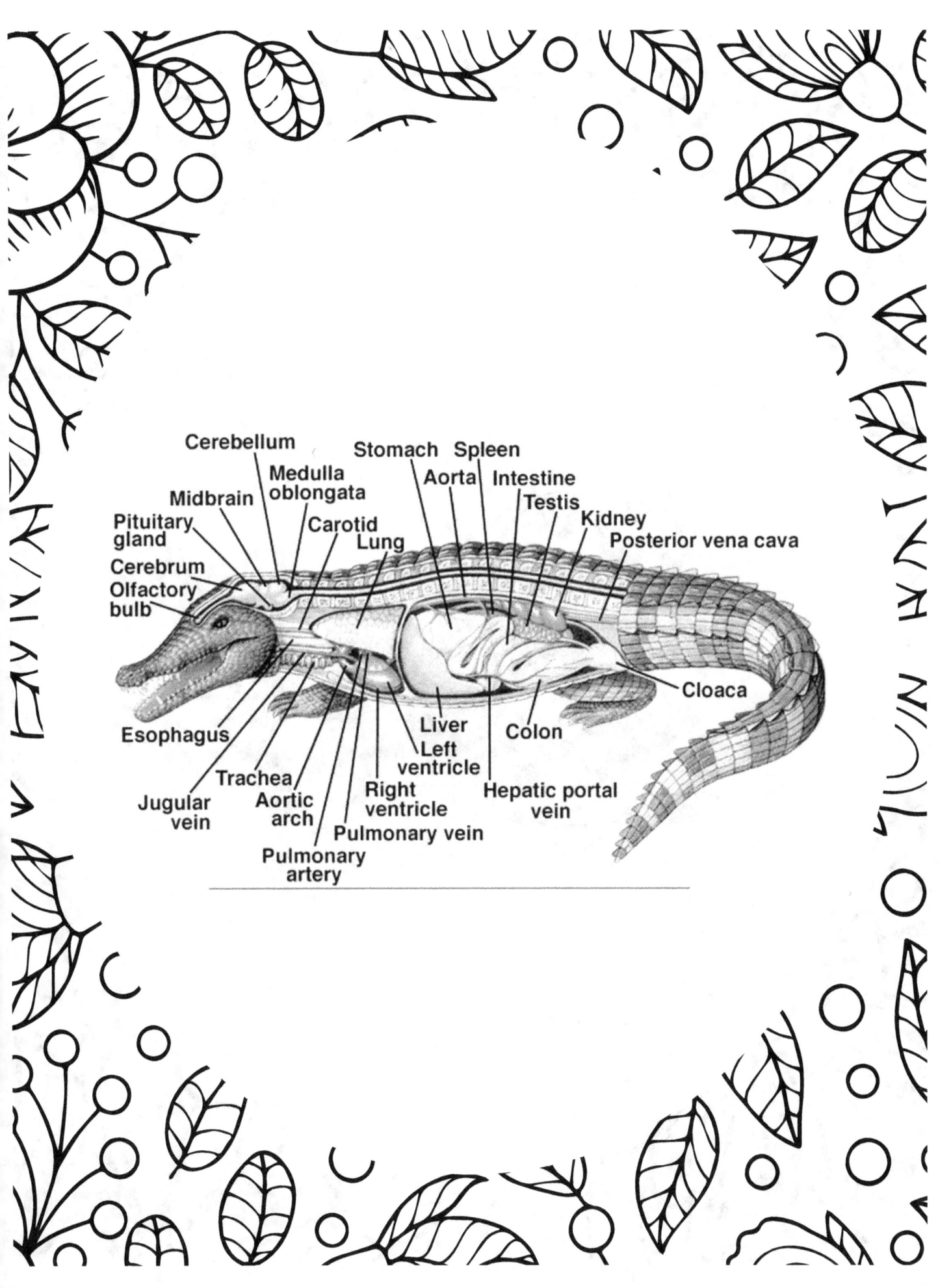

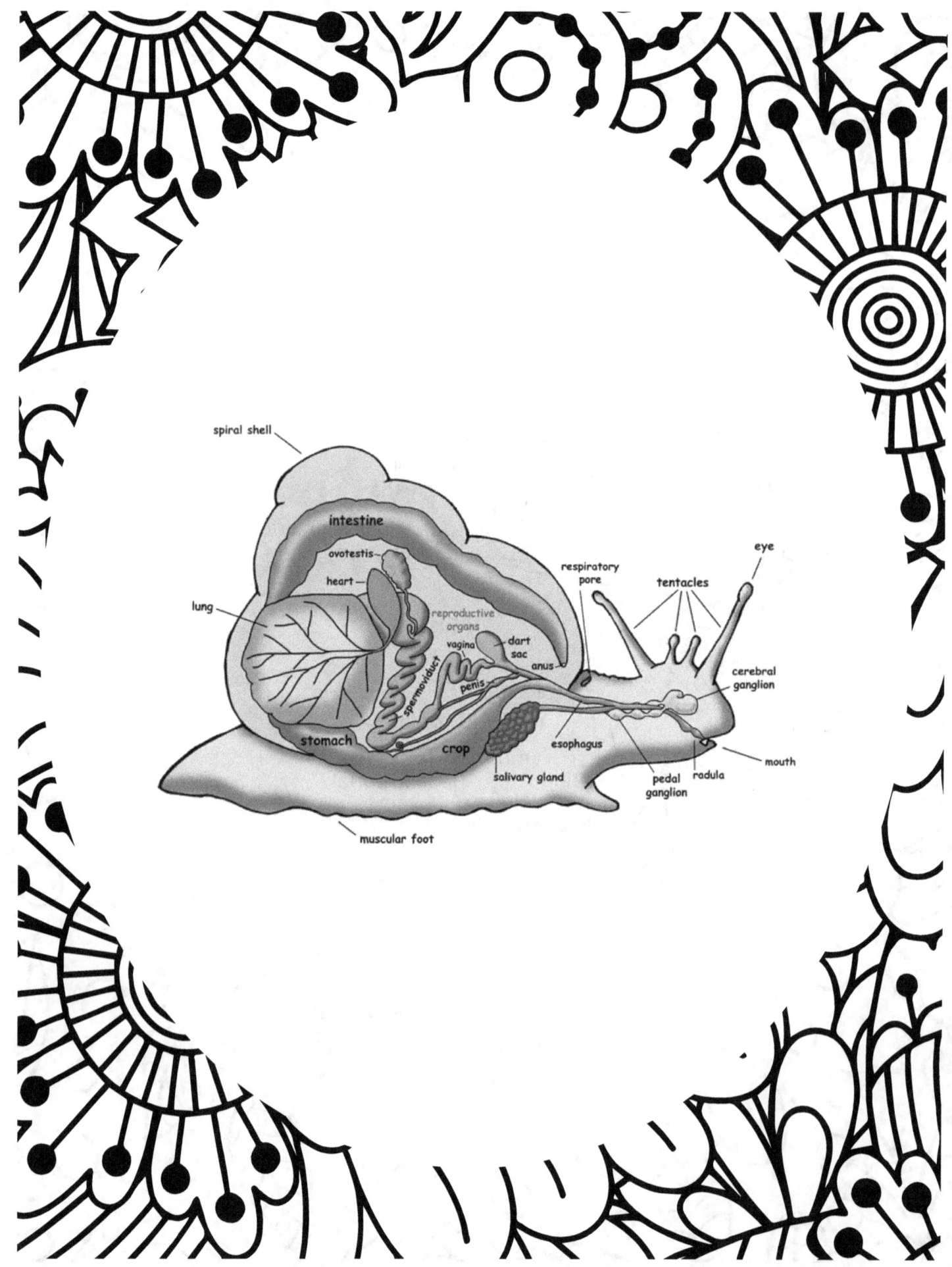

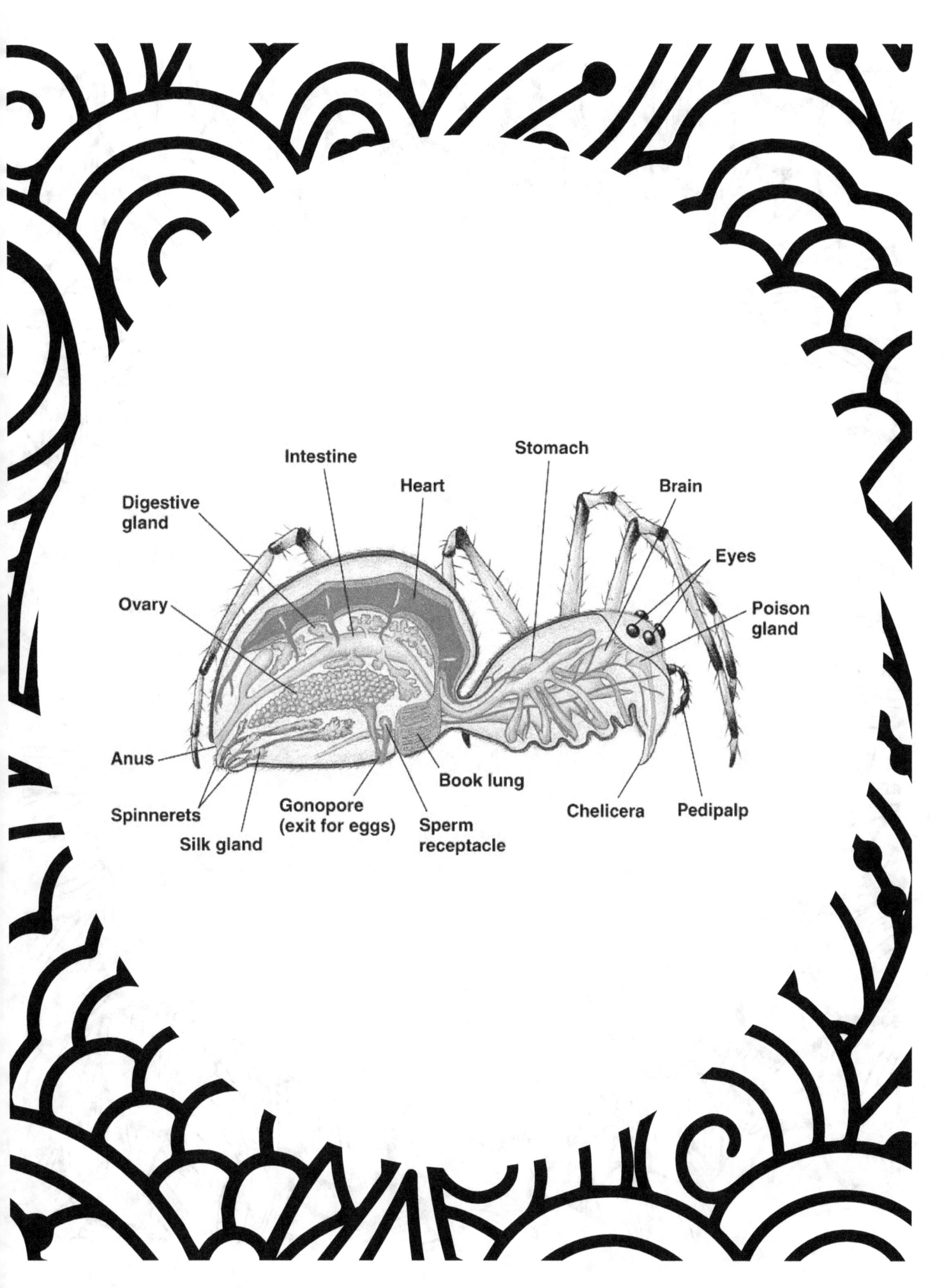

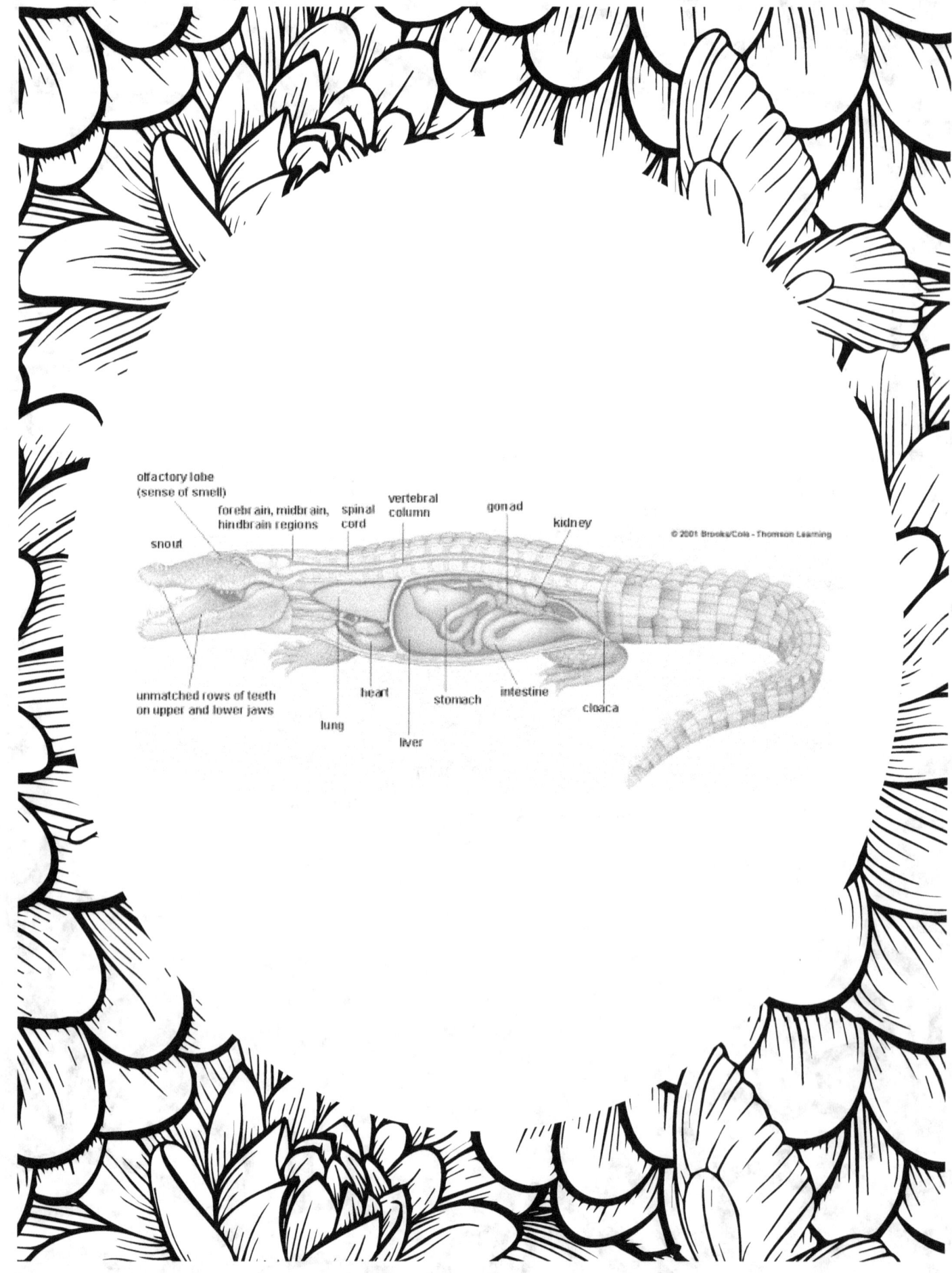

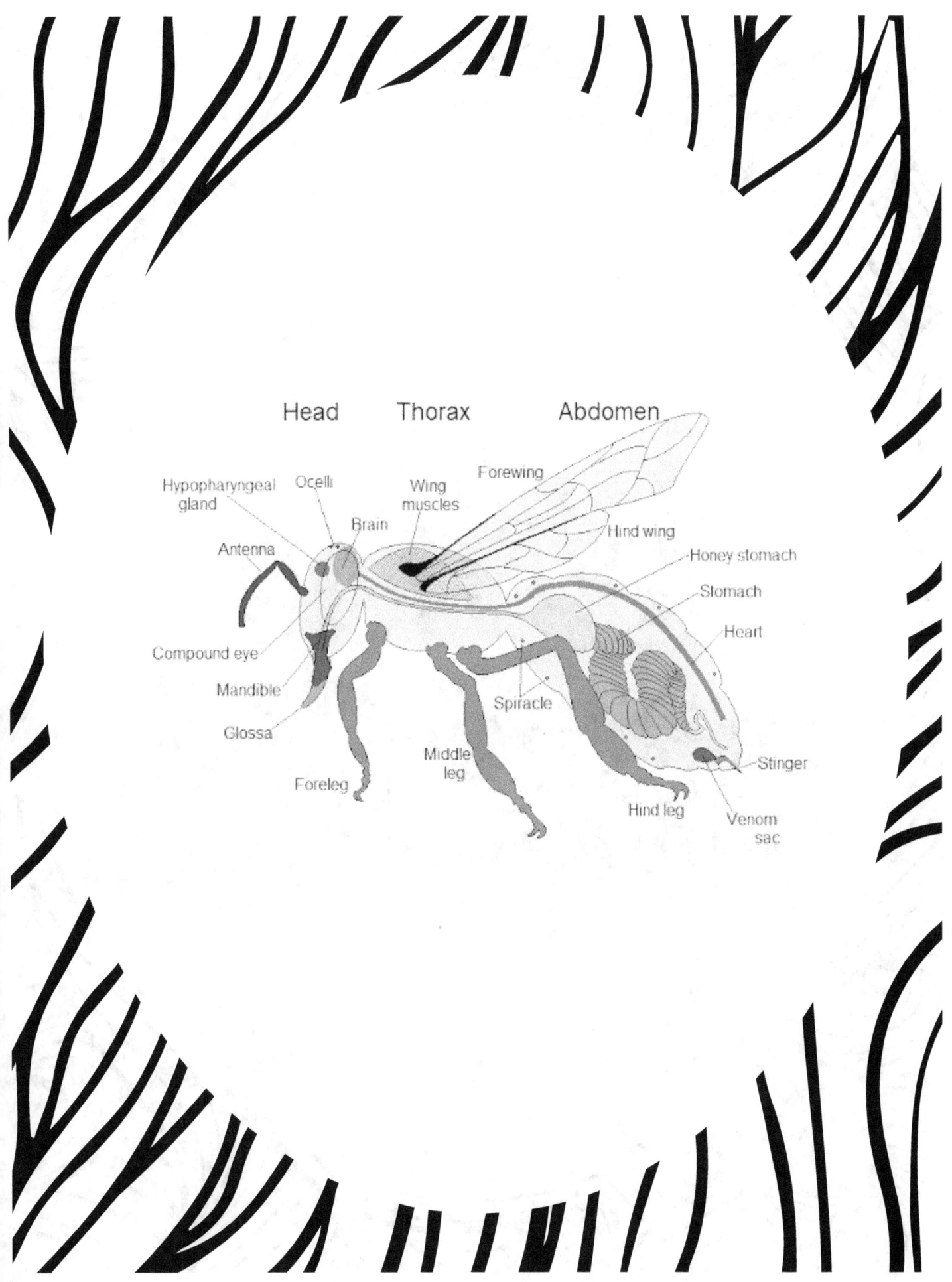

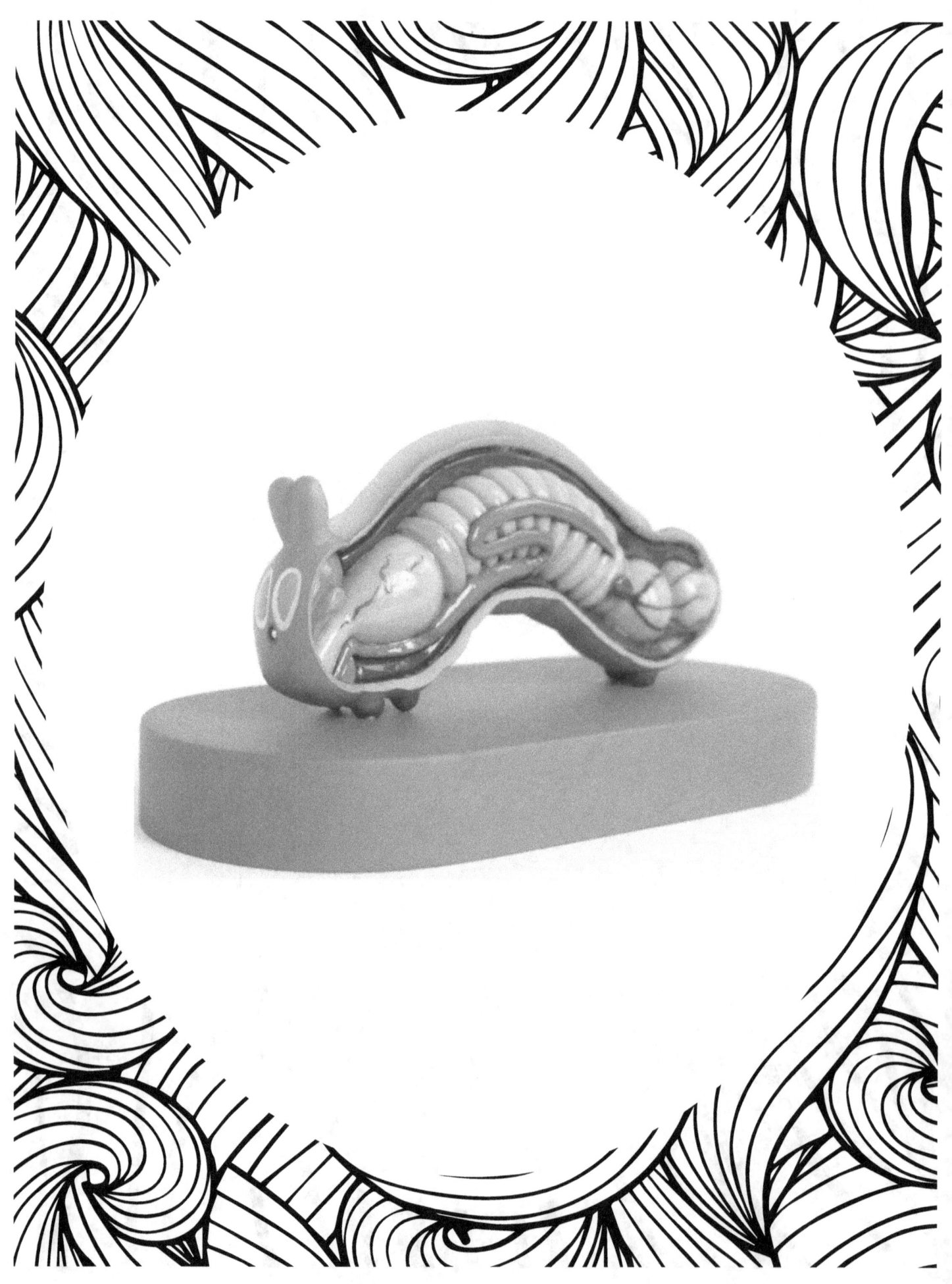

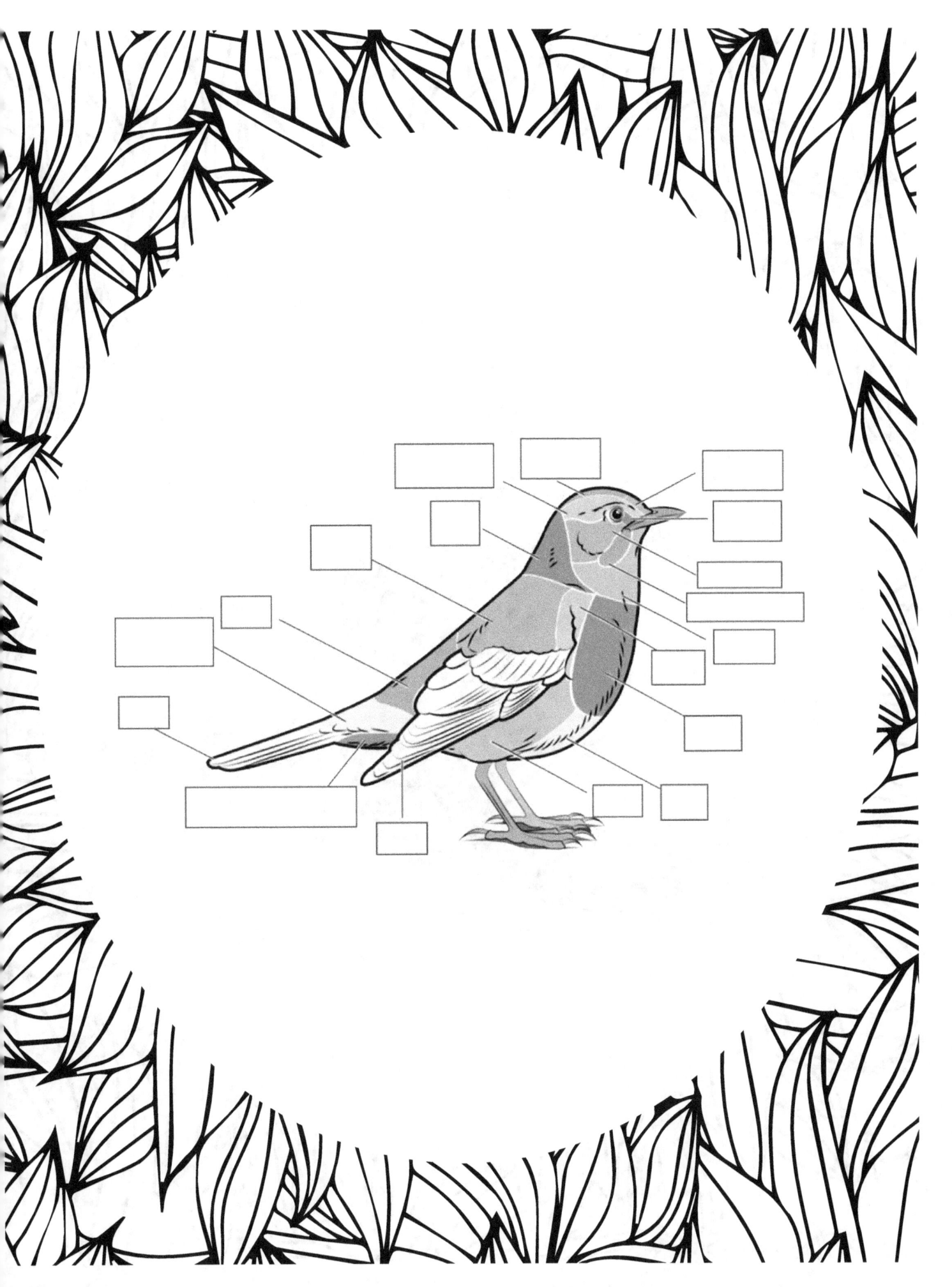

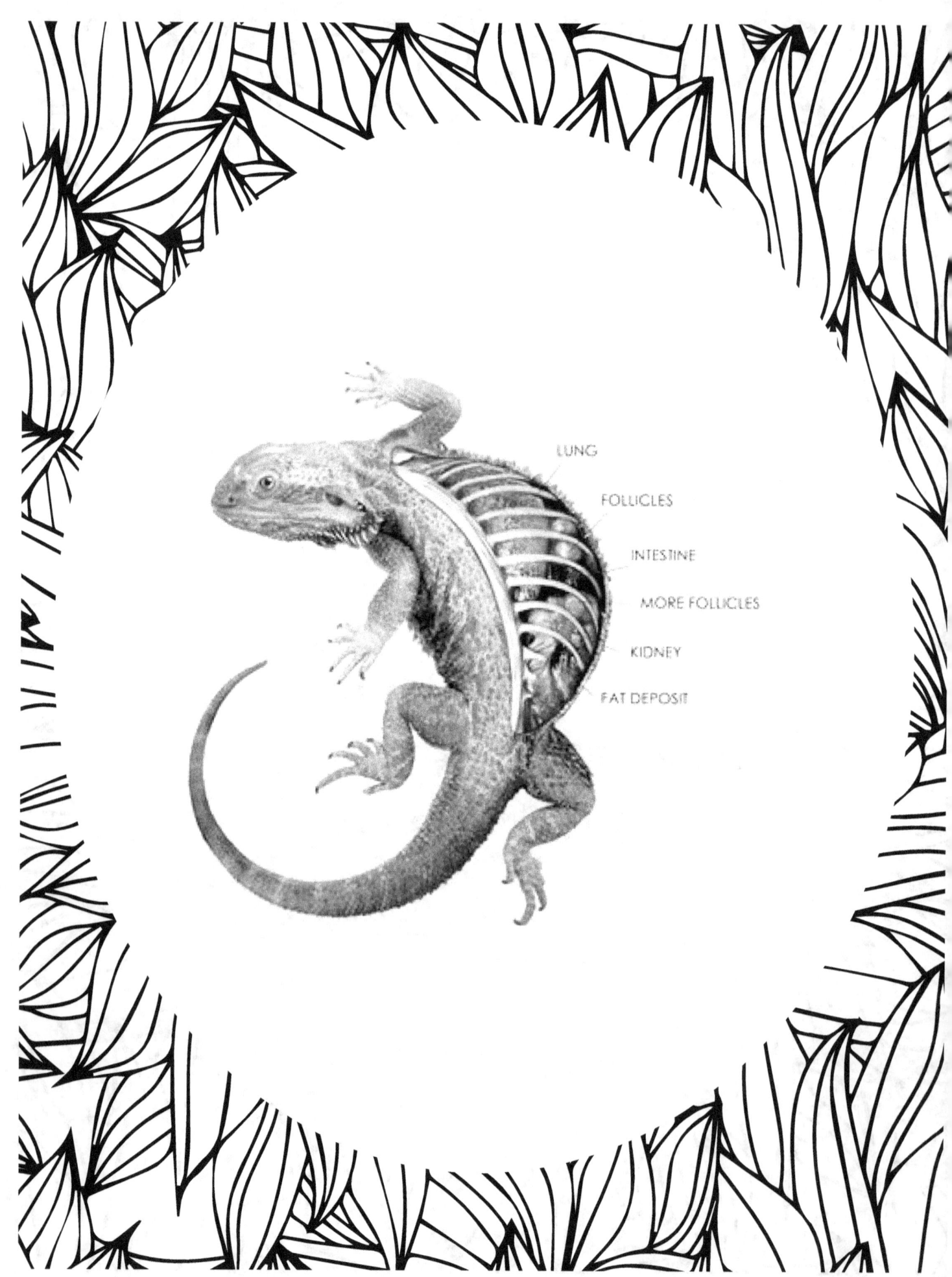

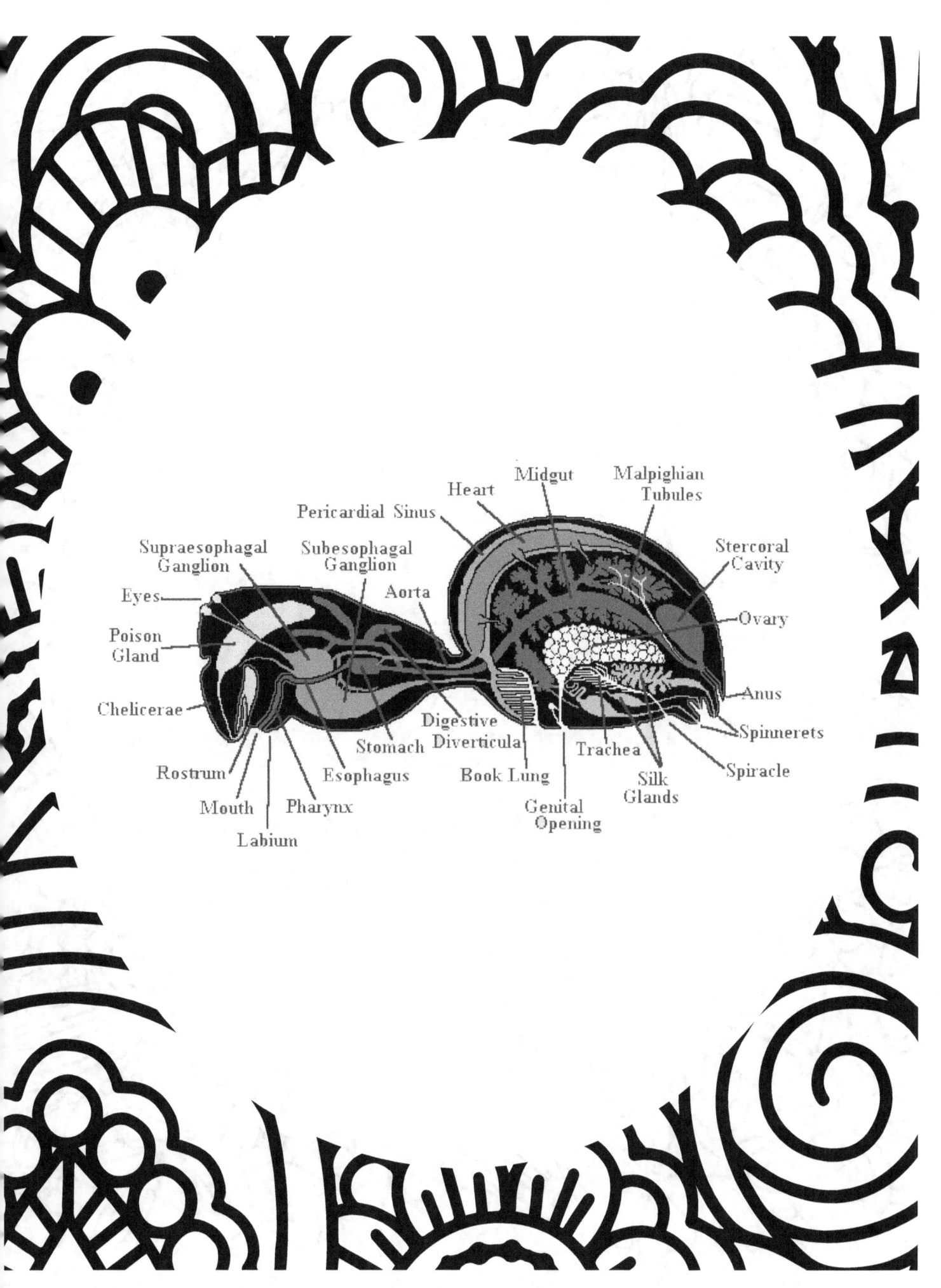

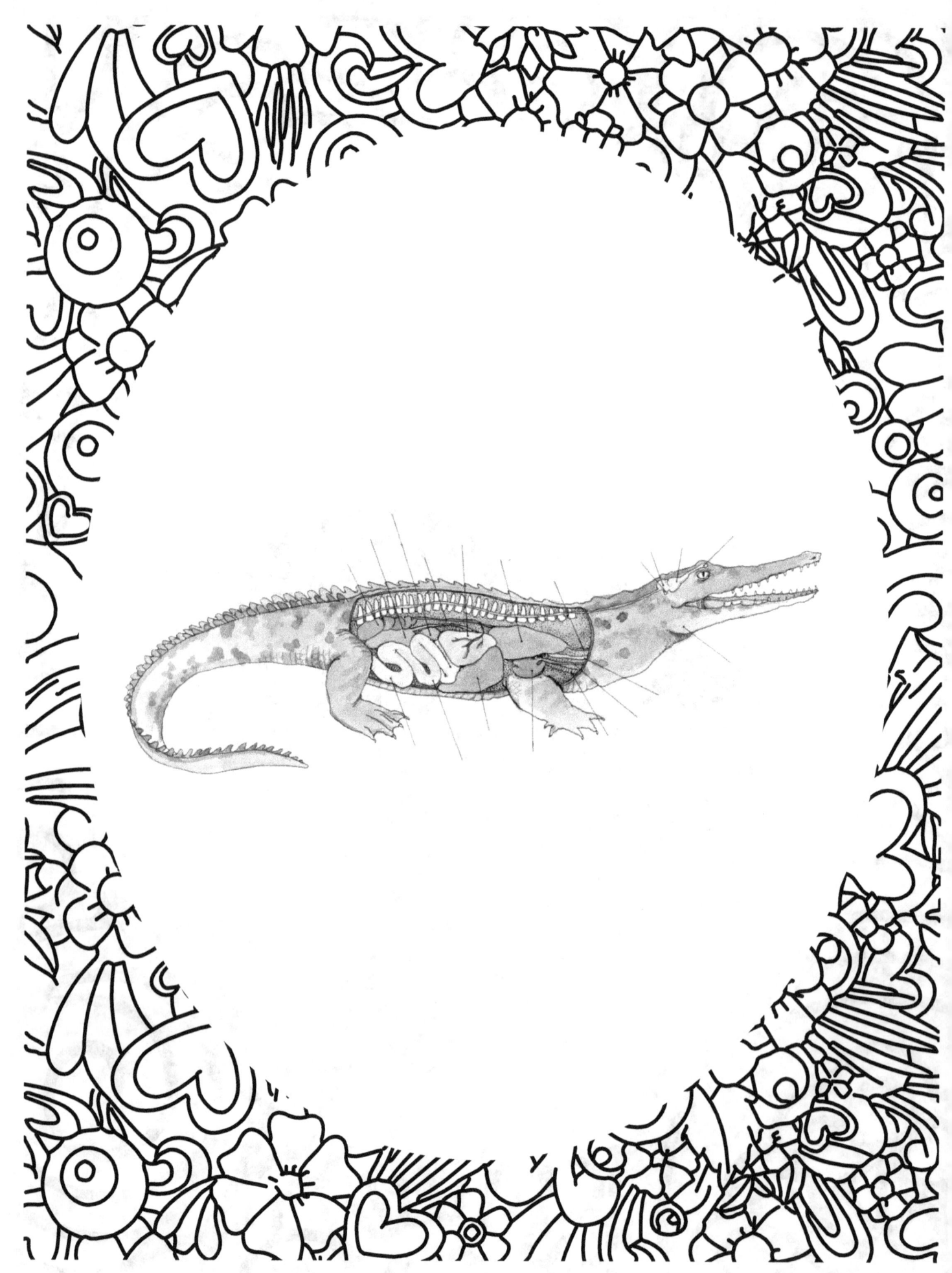

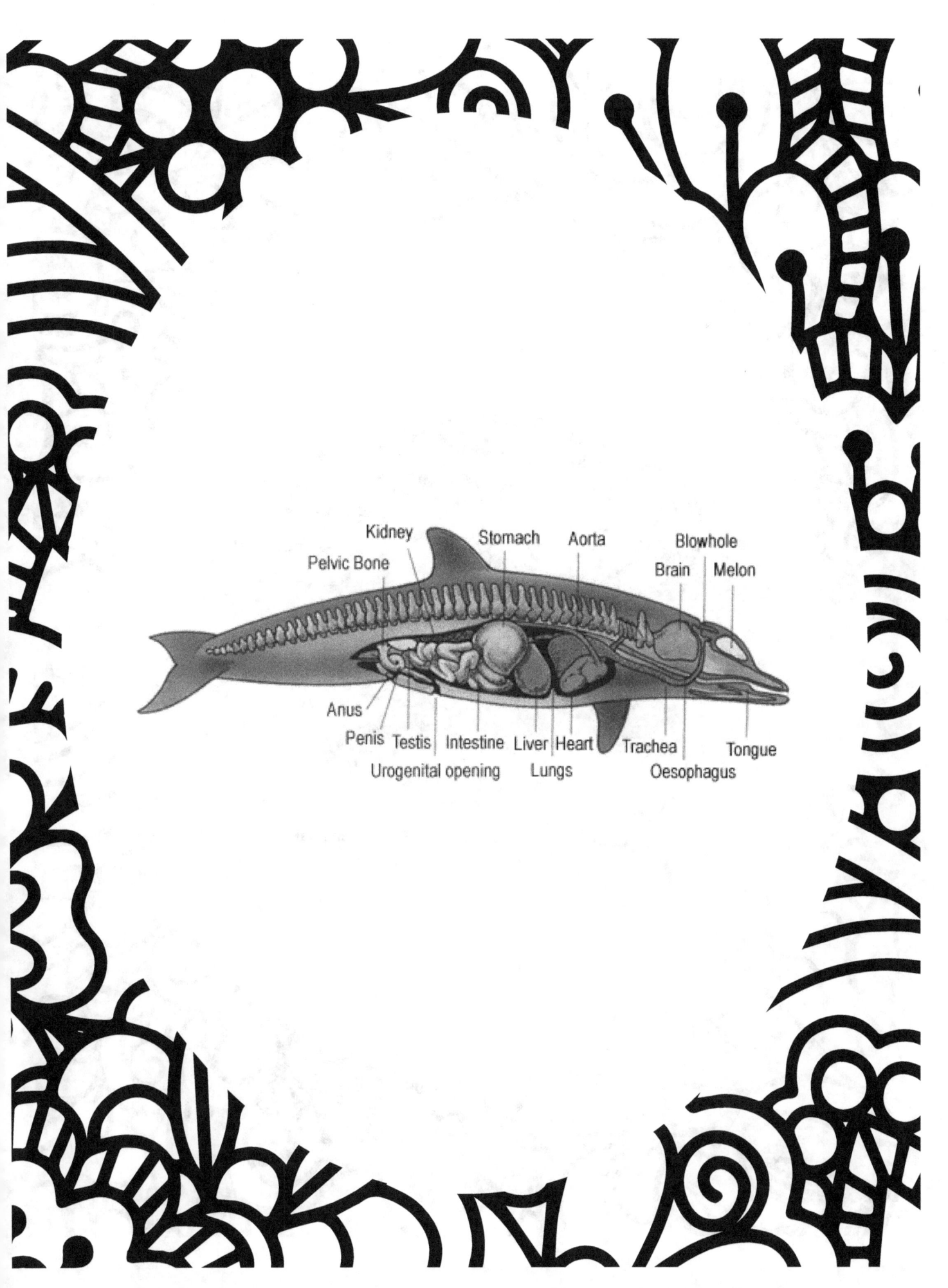

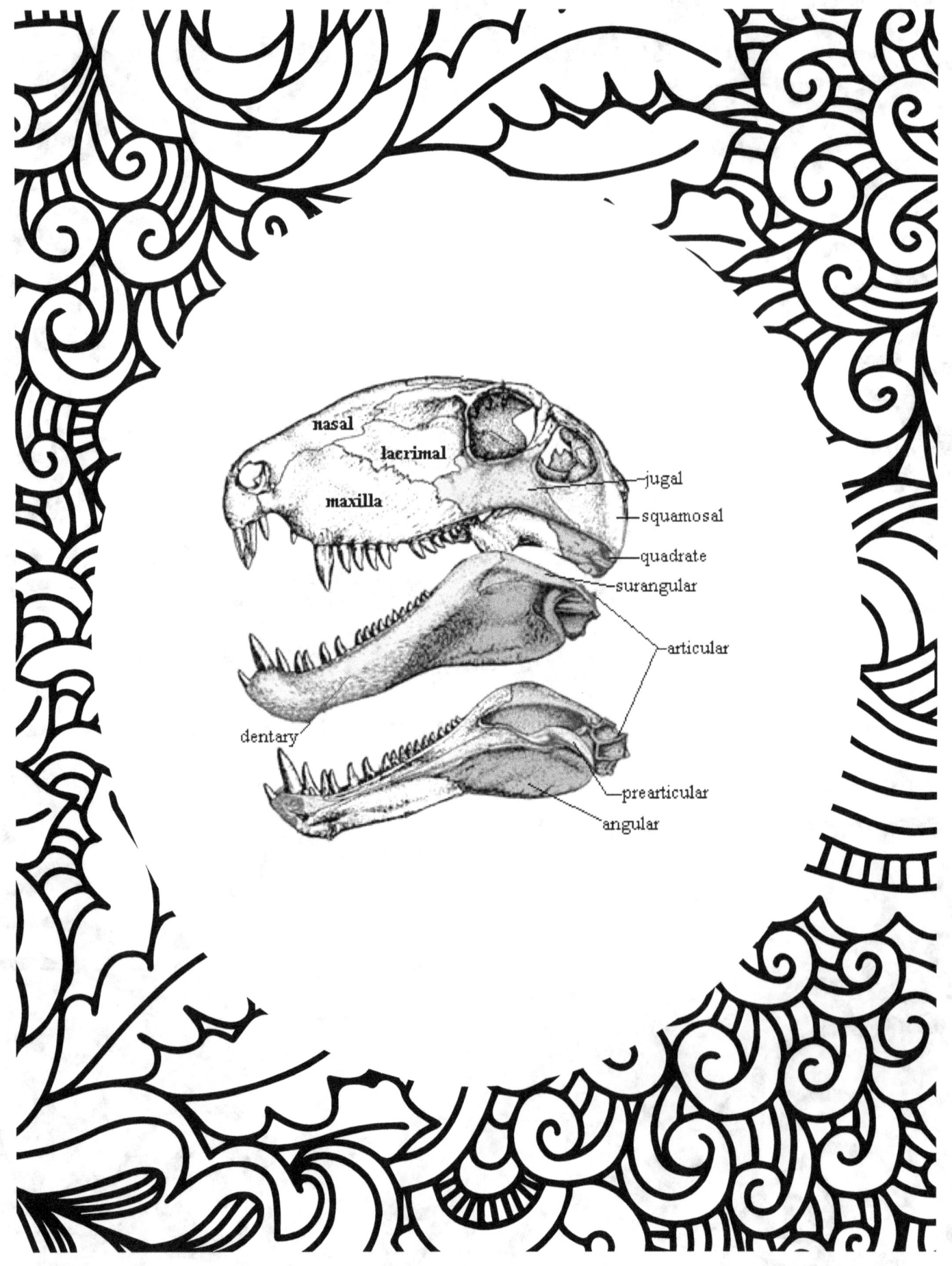

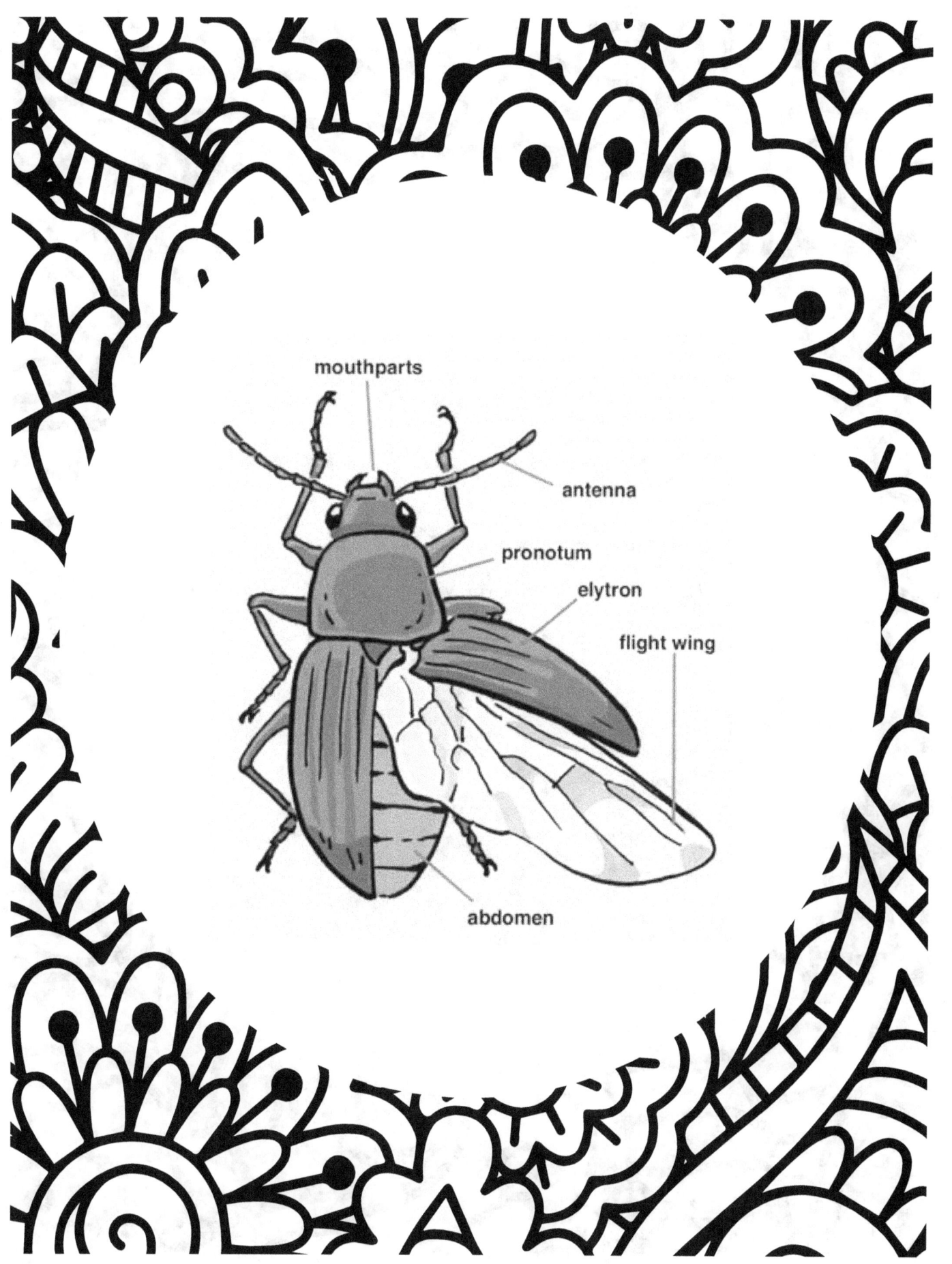

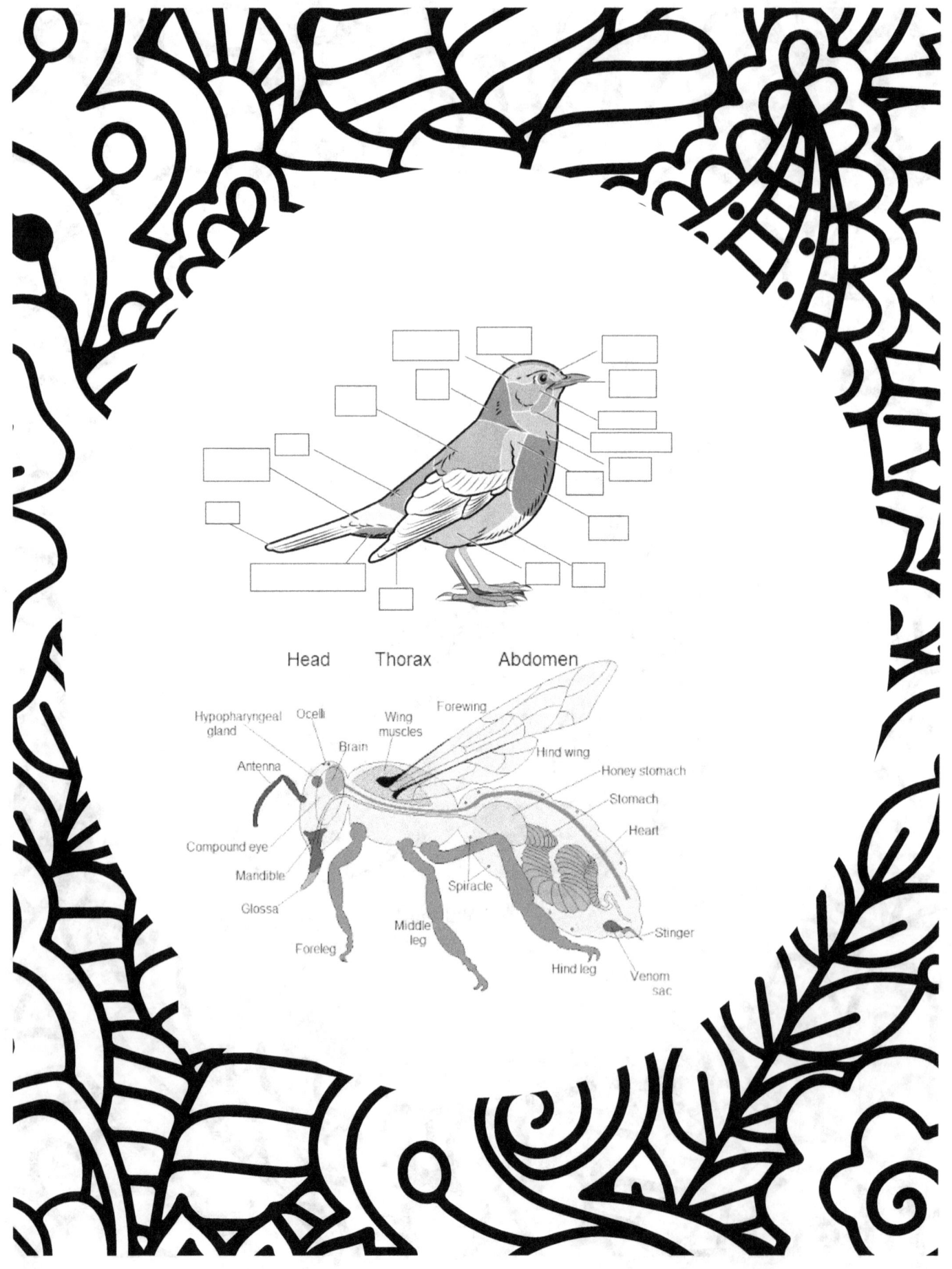

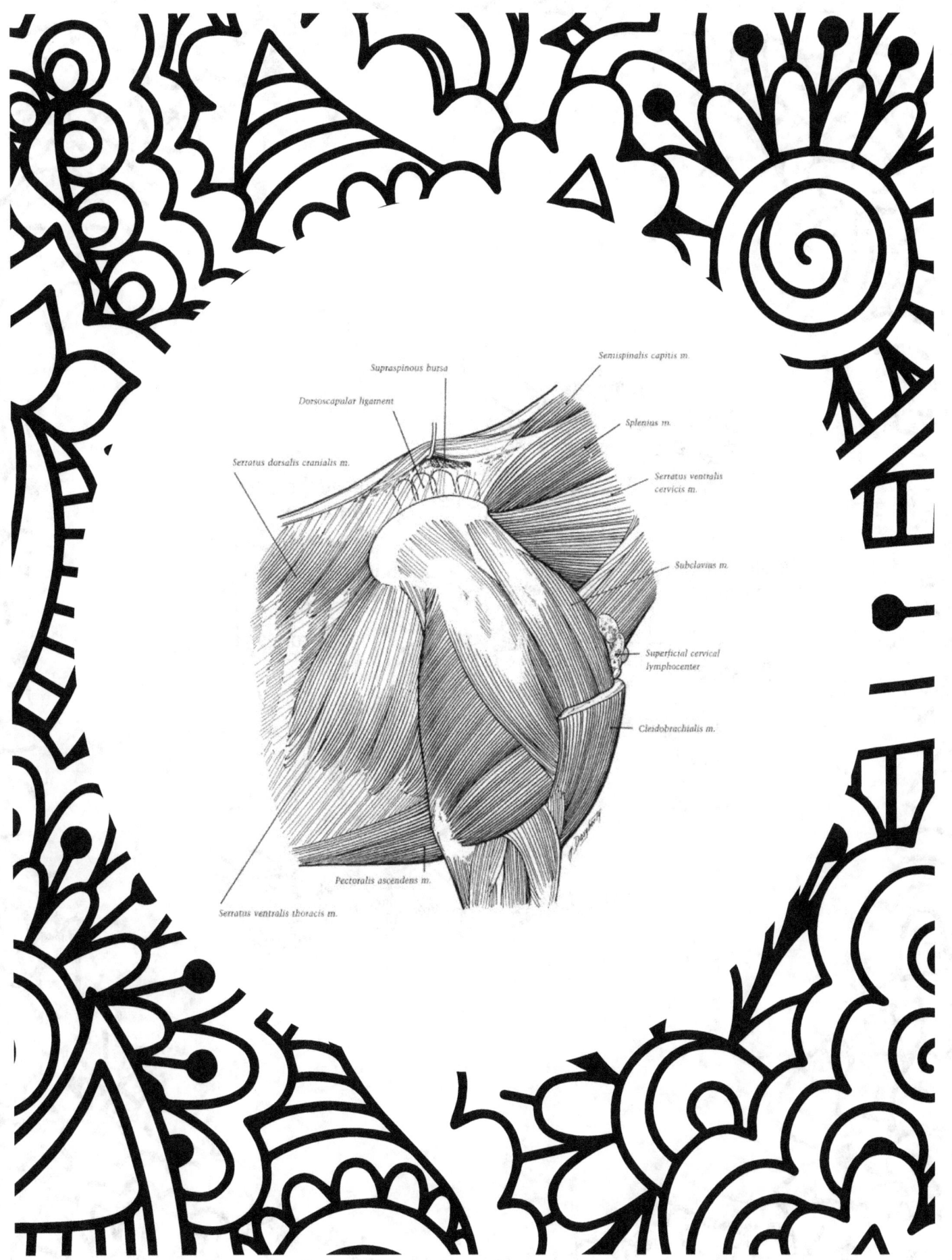

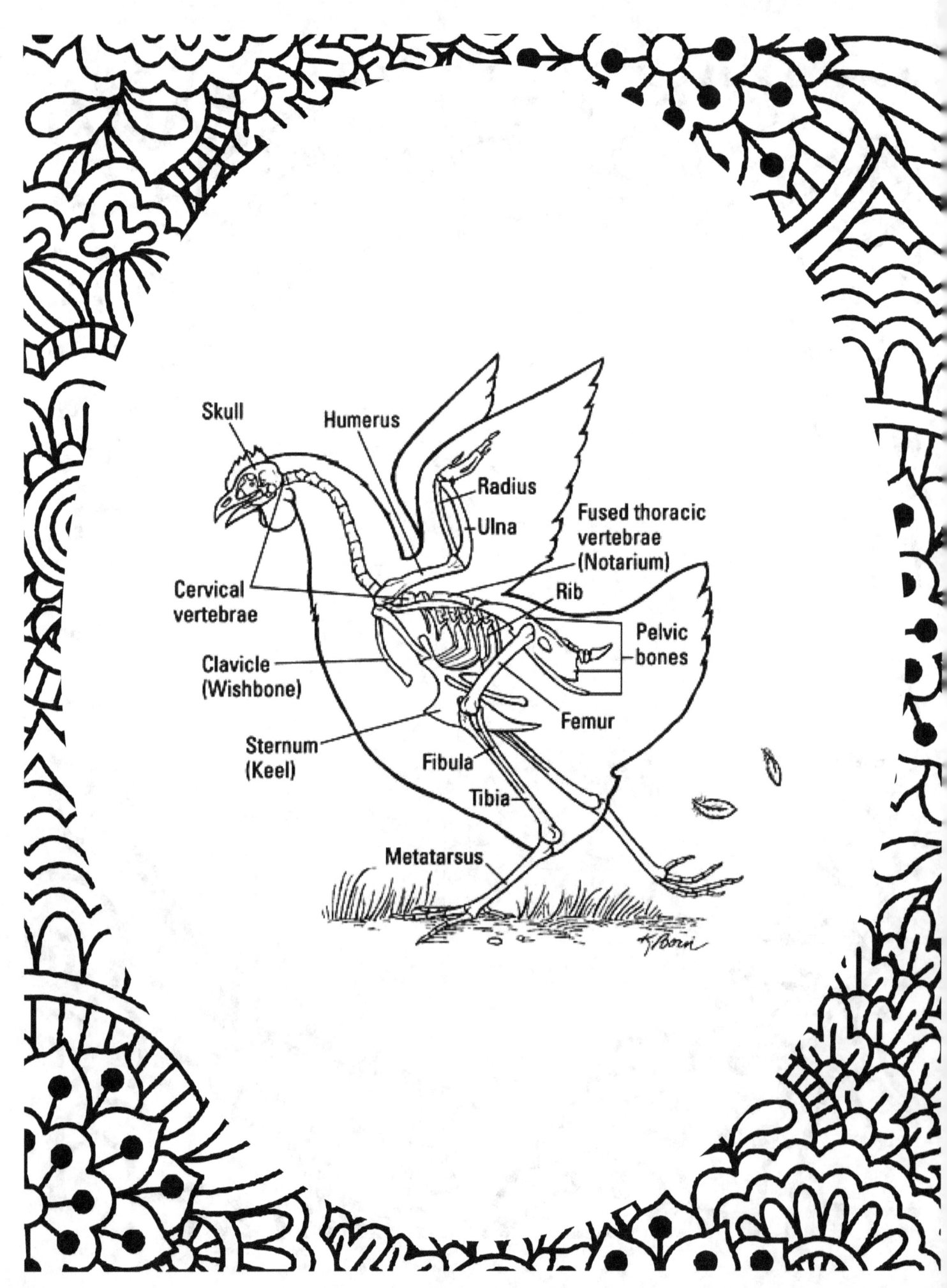

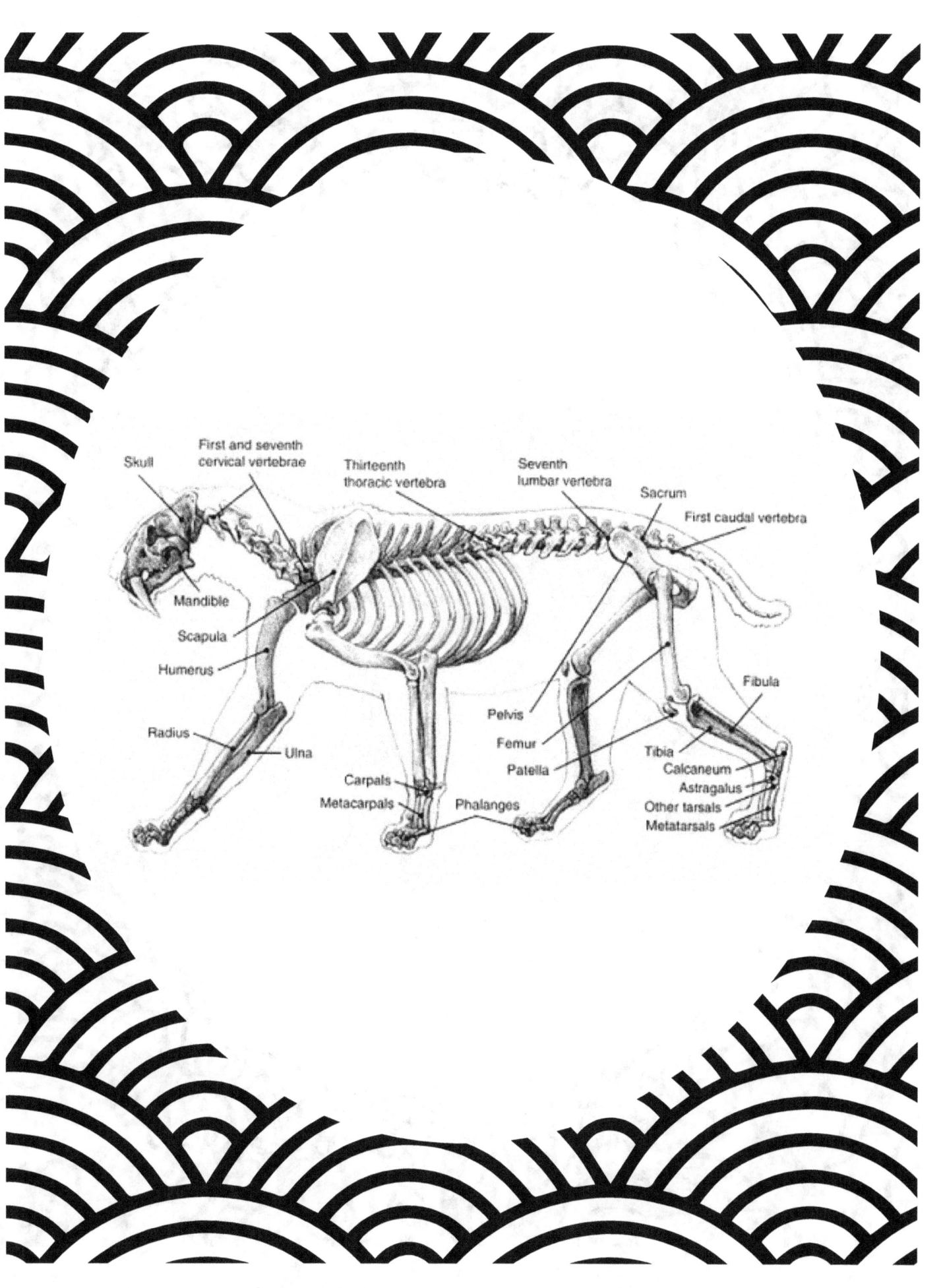

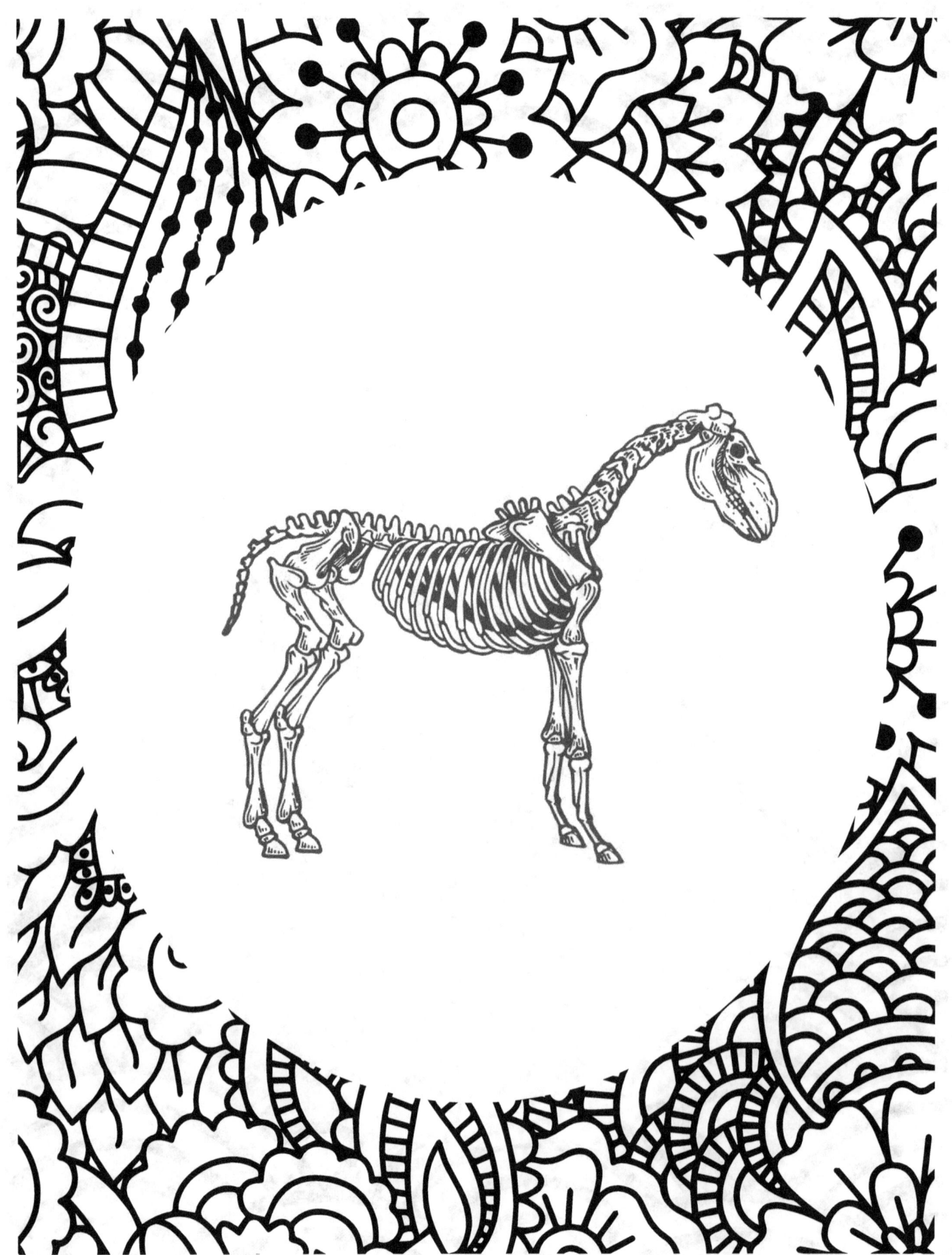

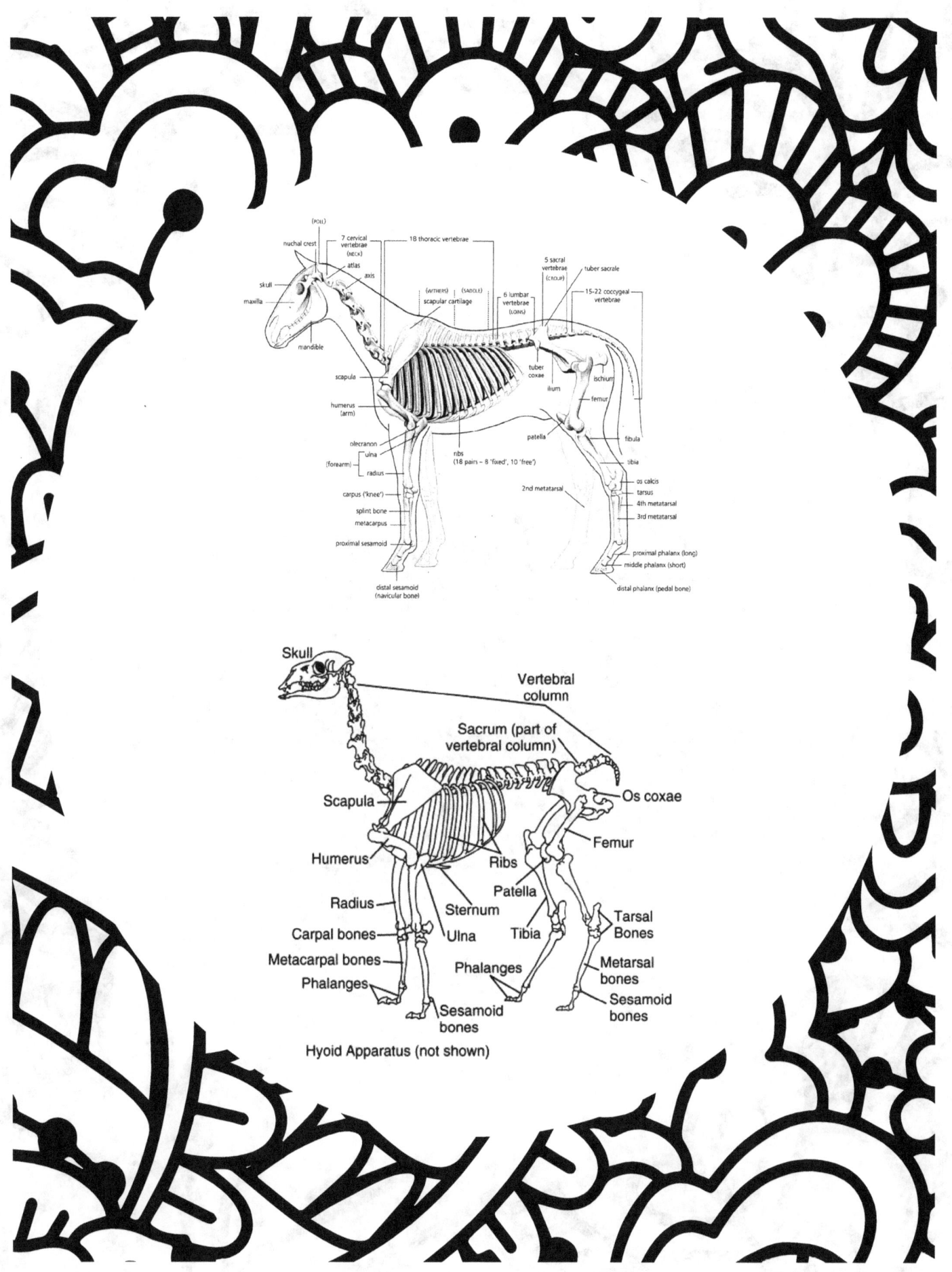

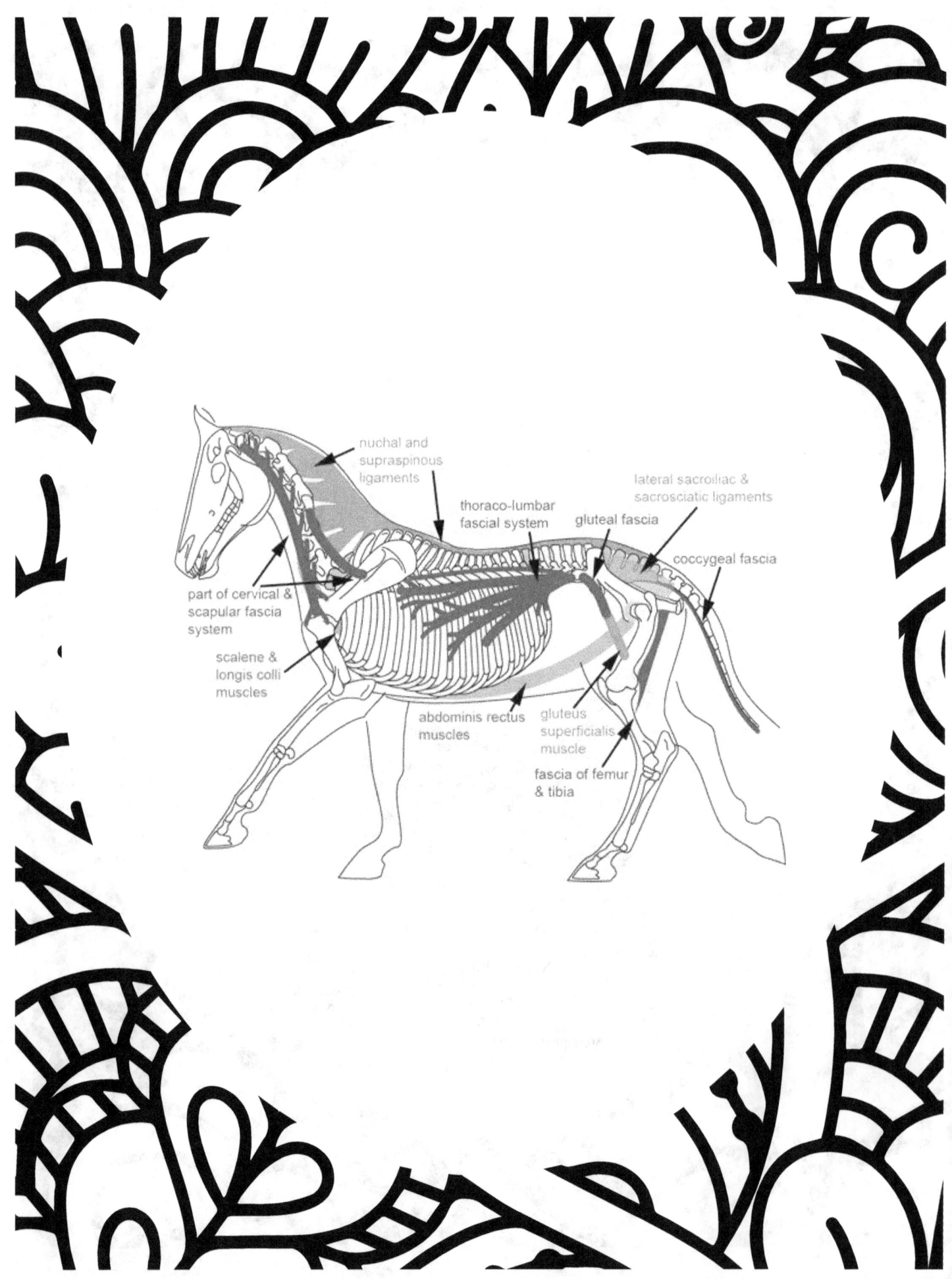

Dinosaur osteology primer (learn the bones!)

Copyright Scott Hartman, 2013.

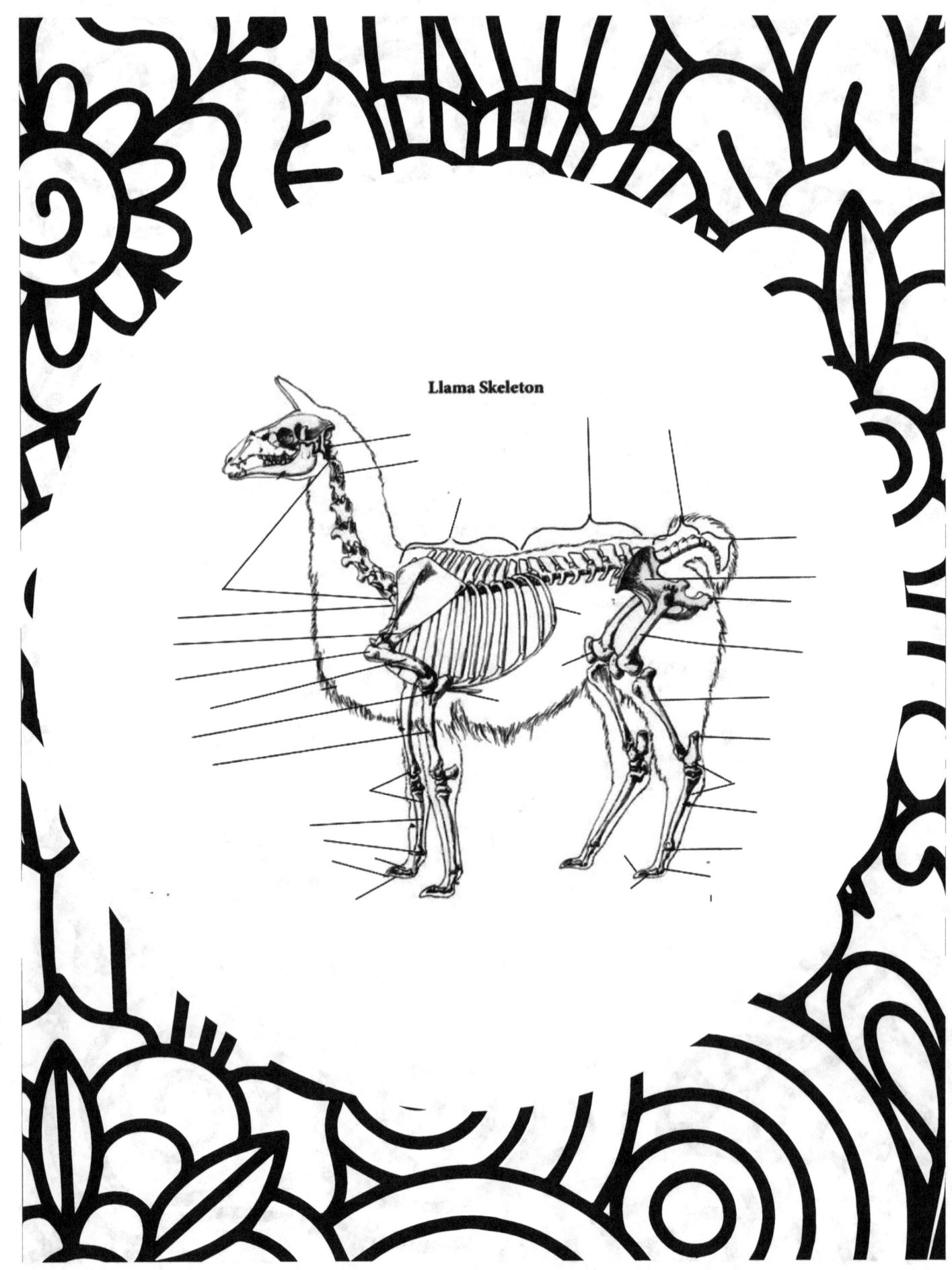

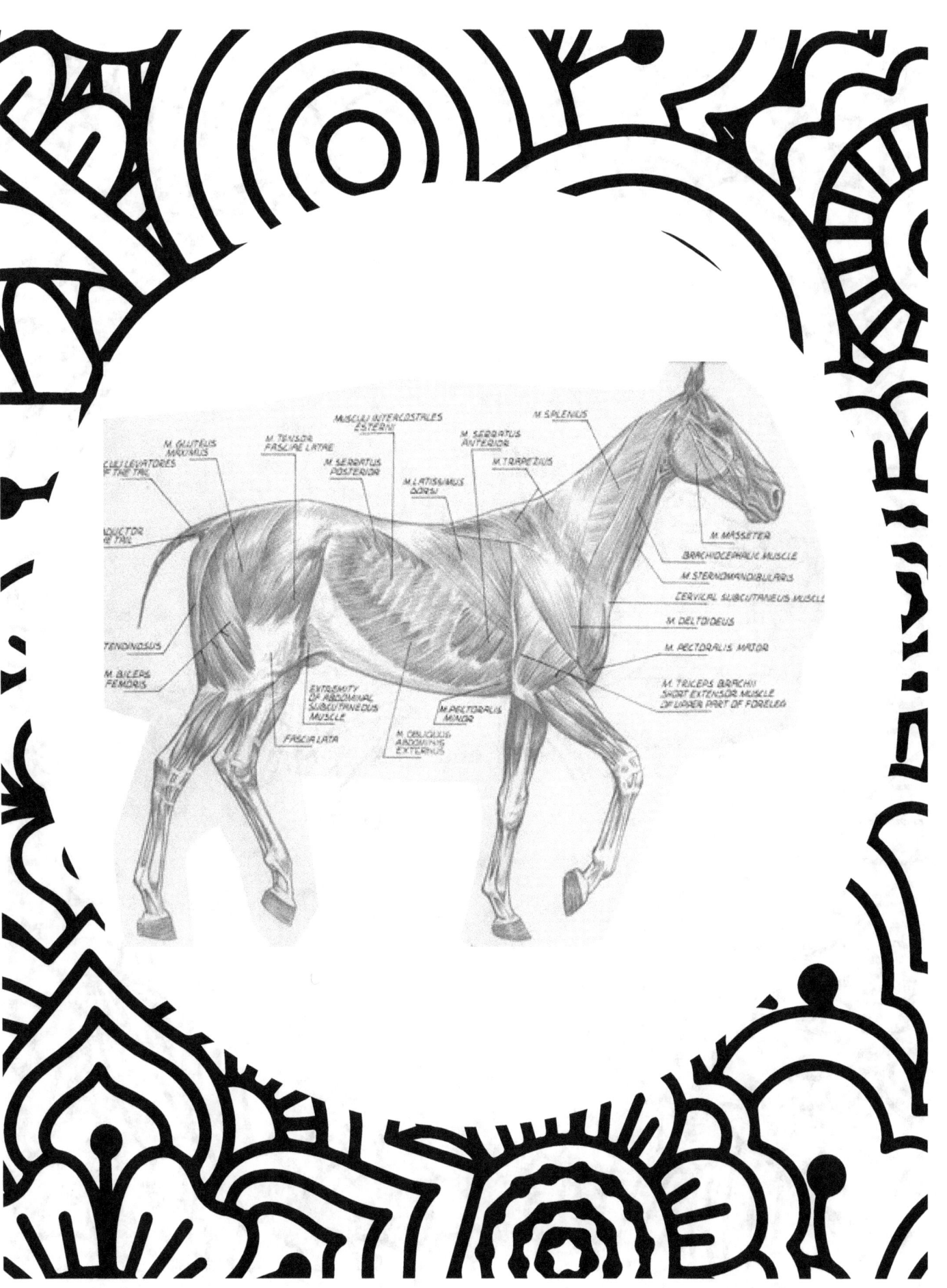

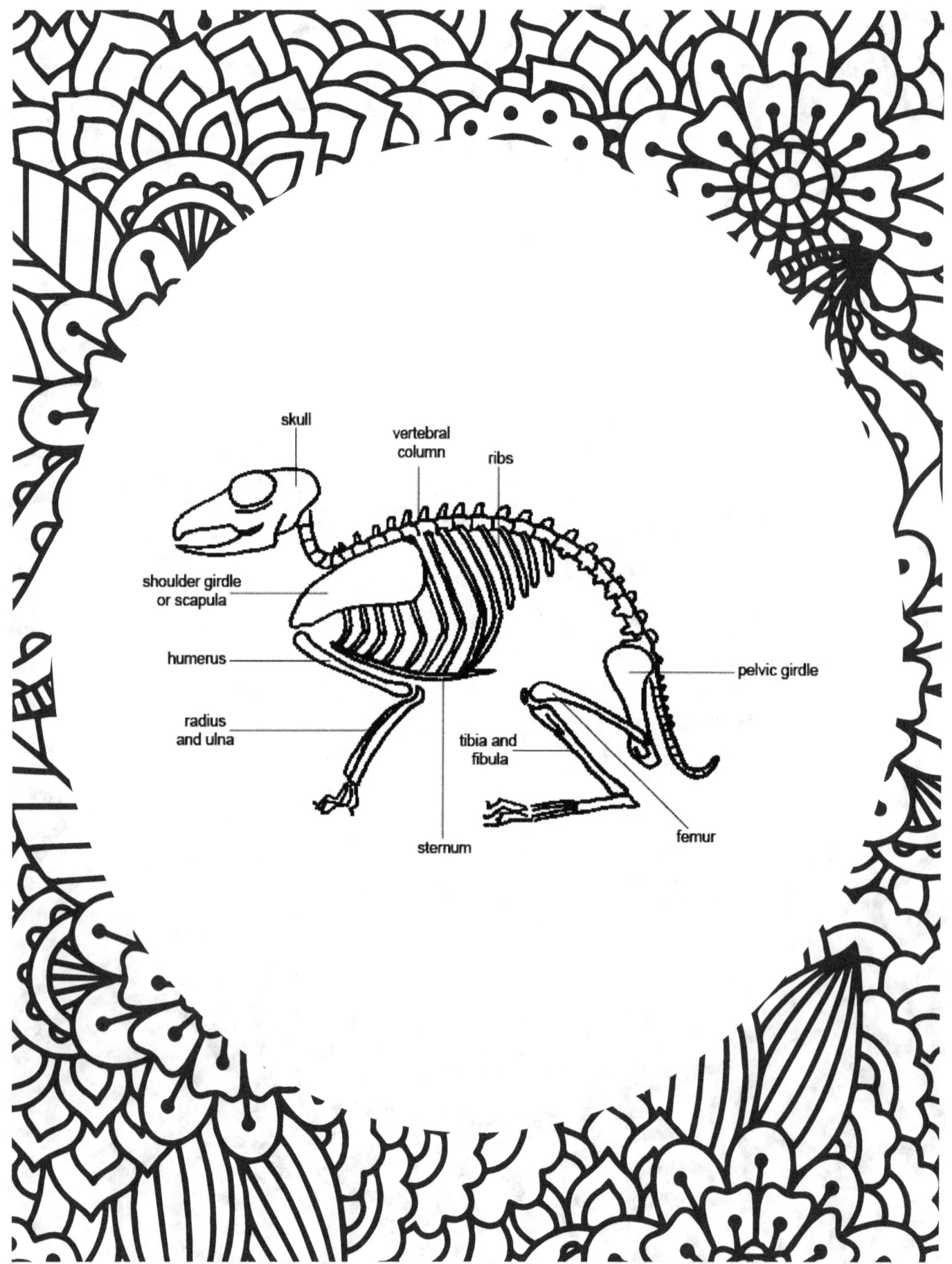

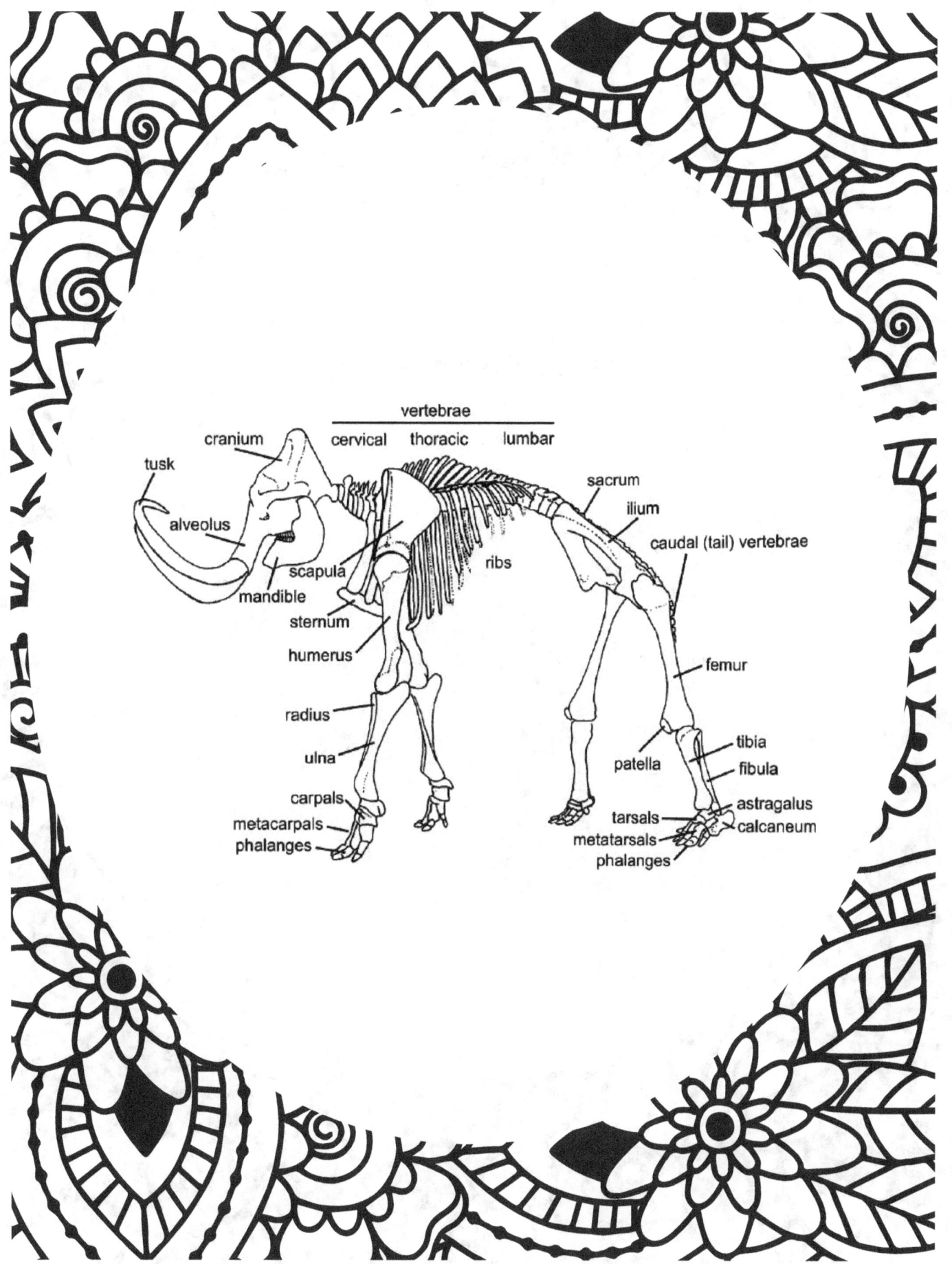

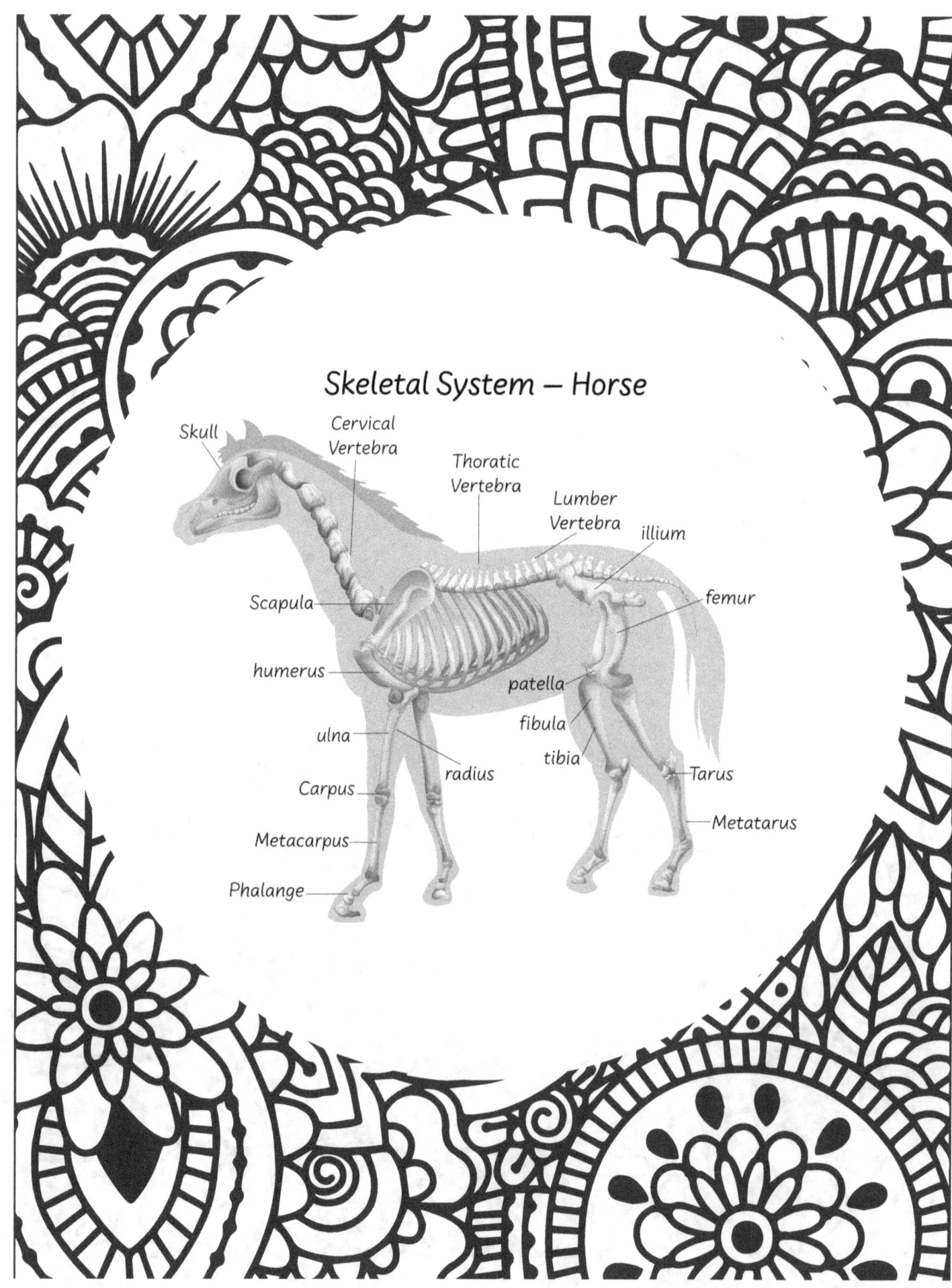

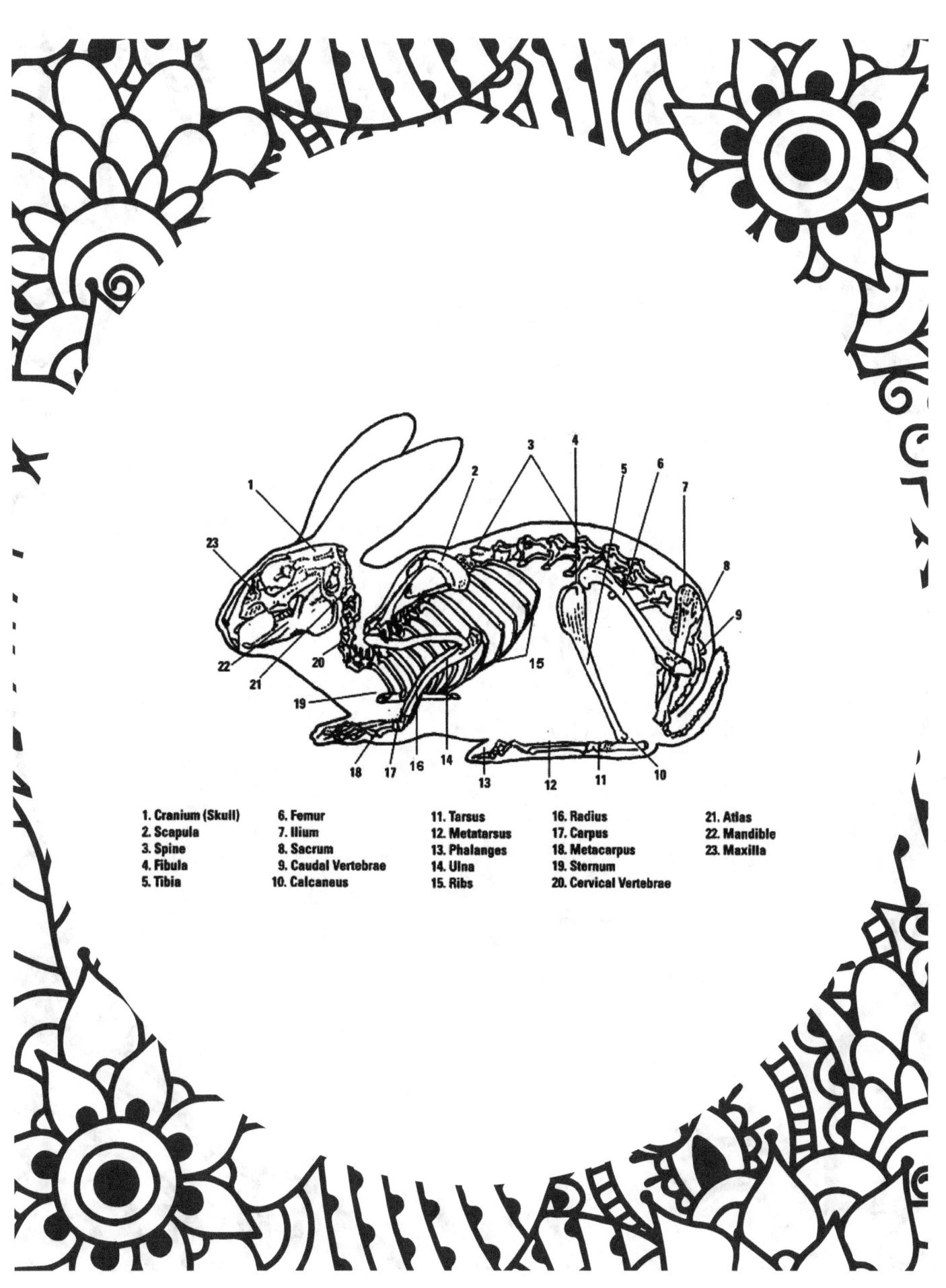

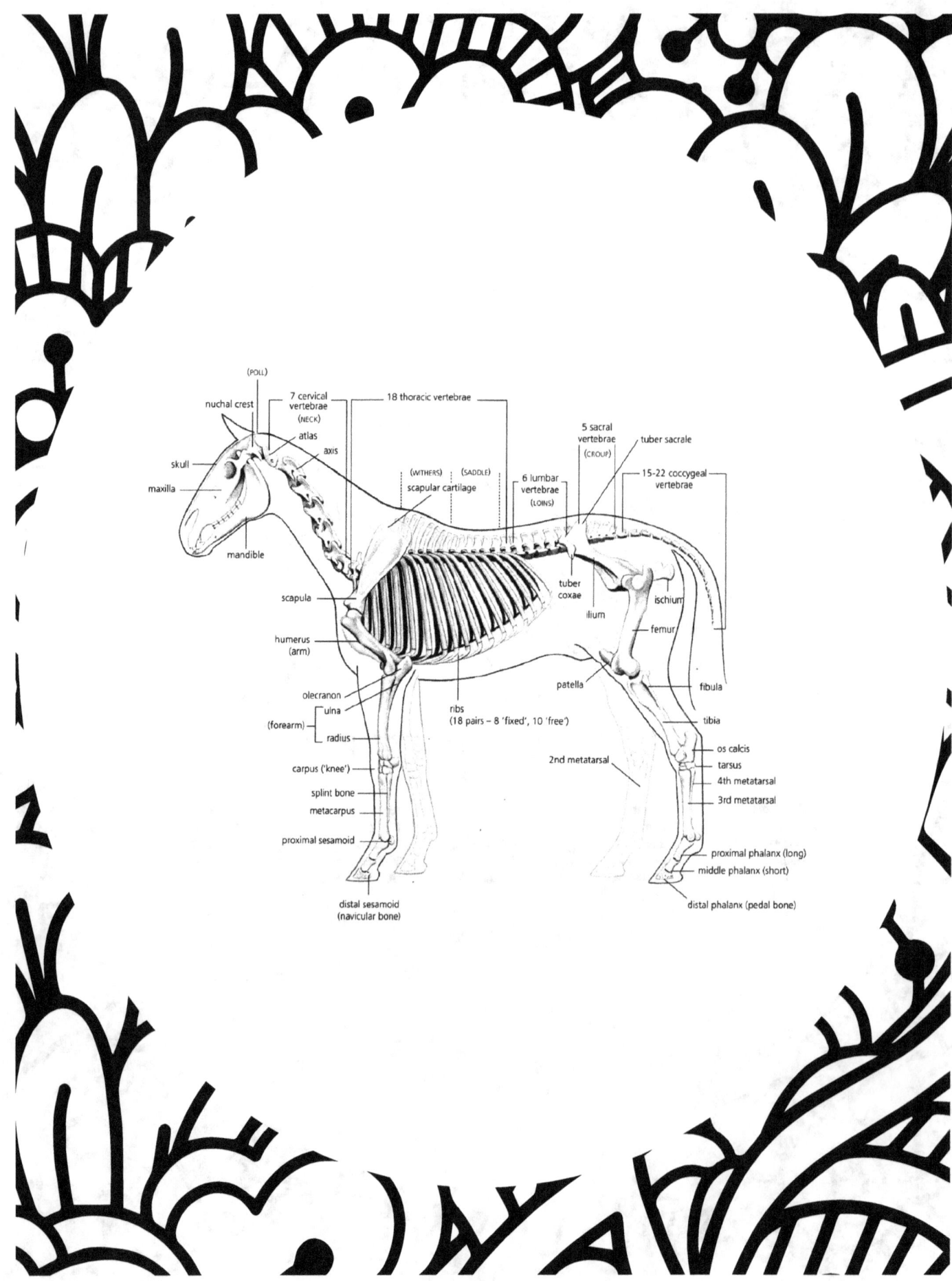

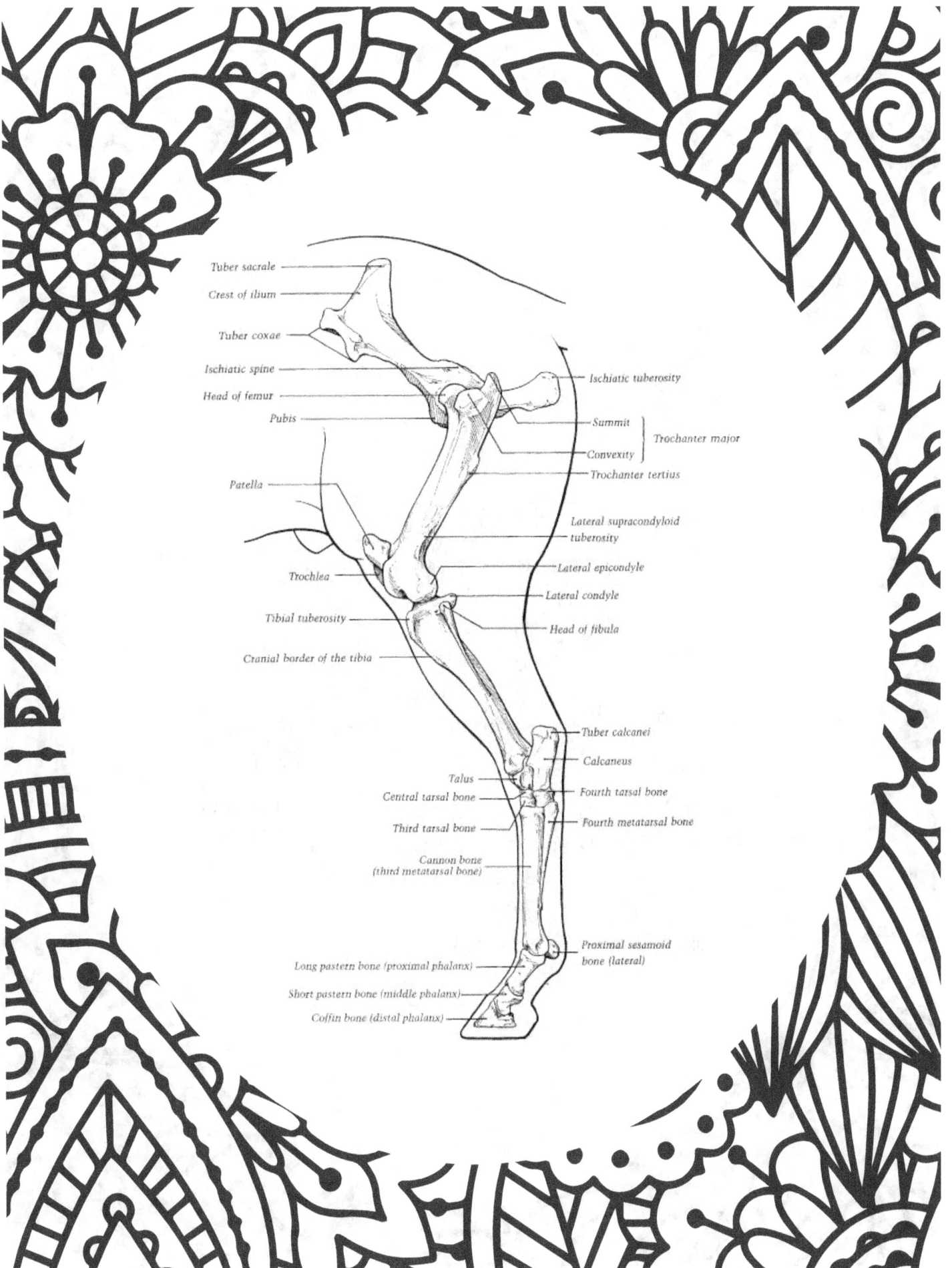

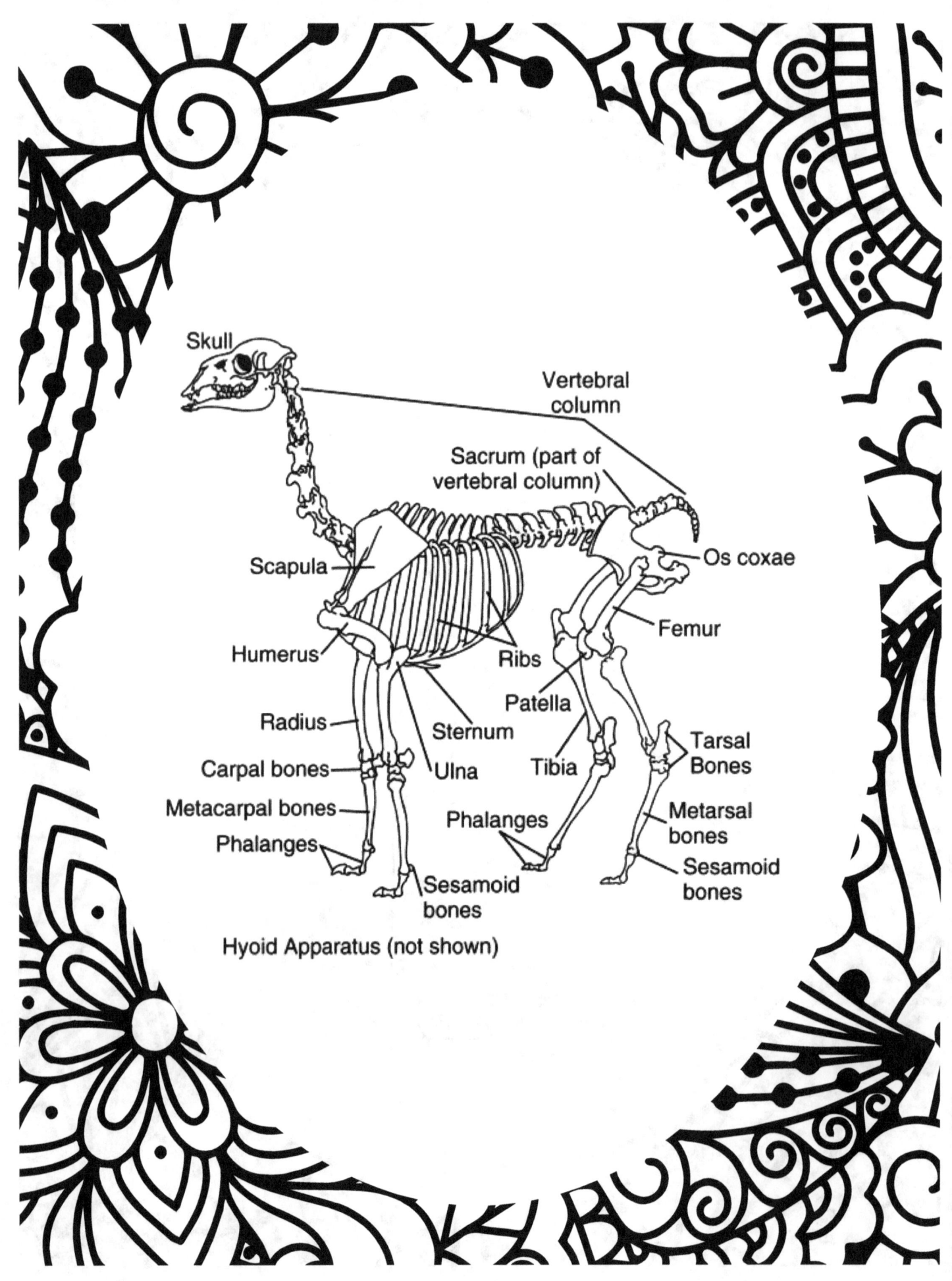

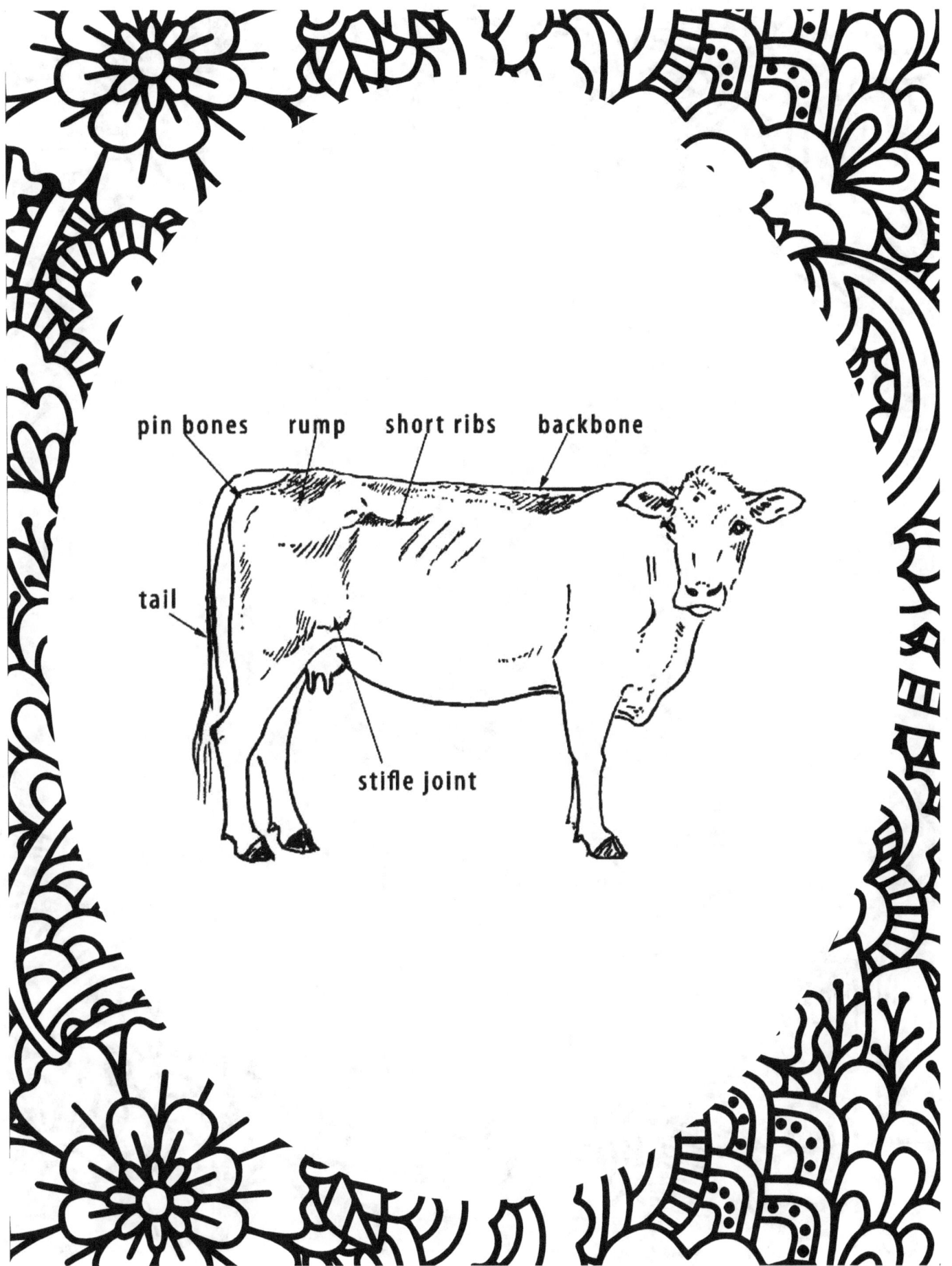

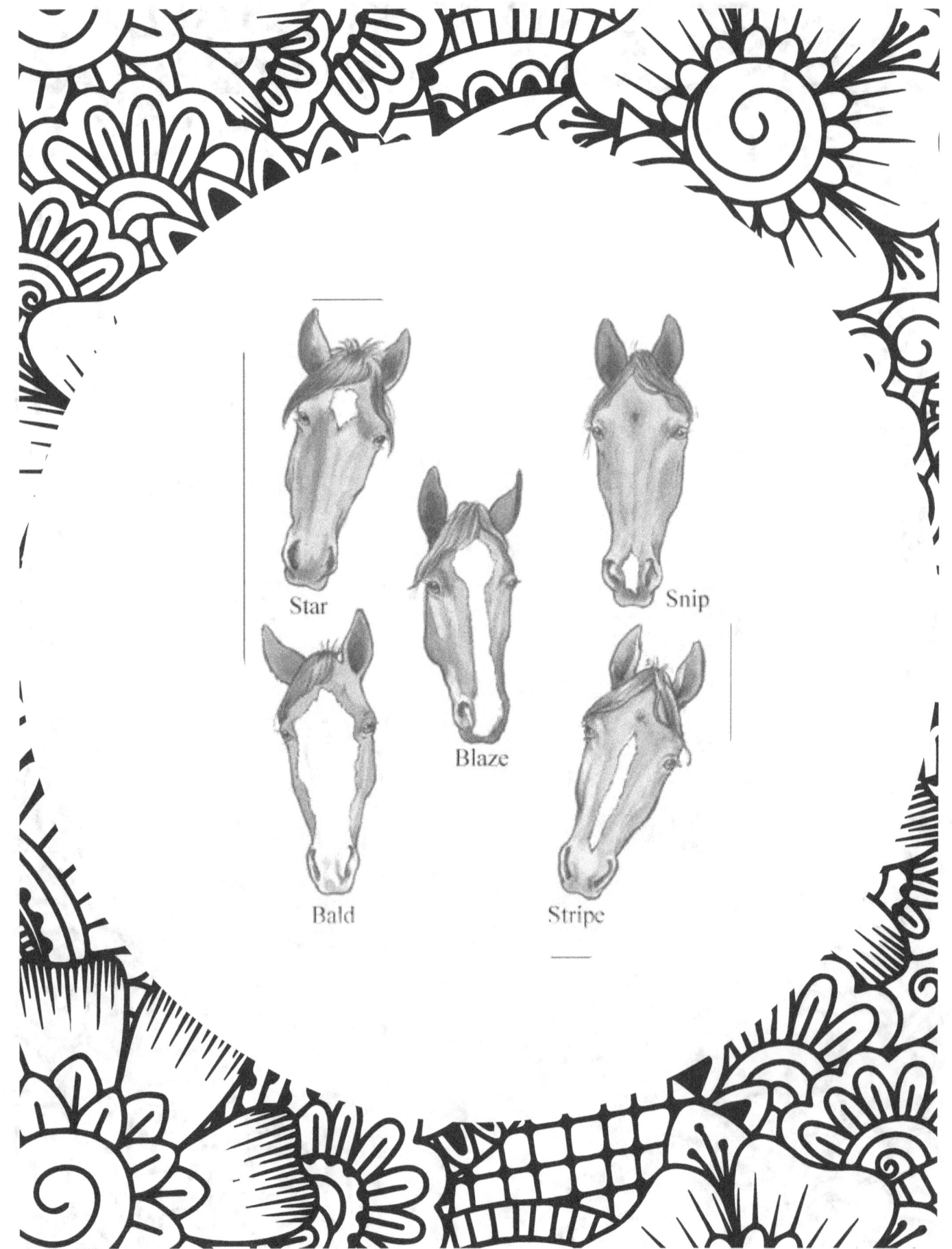

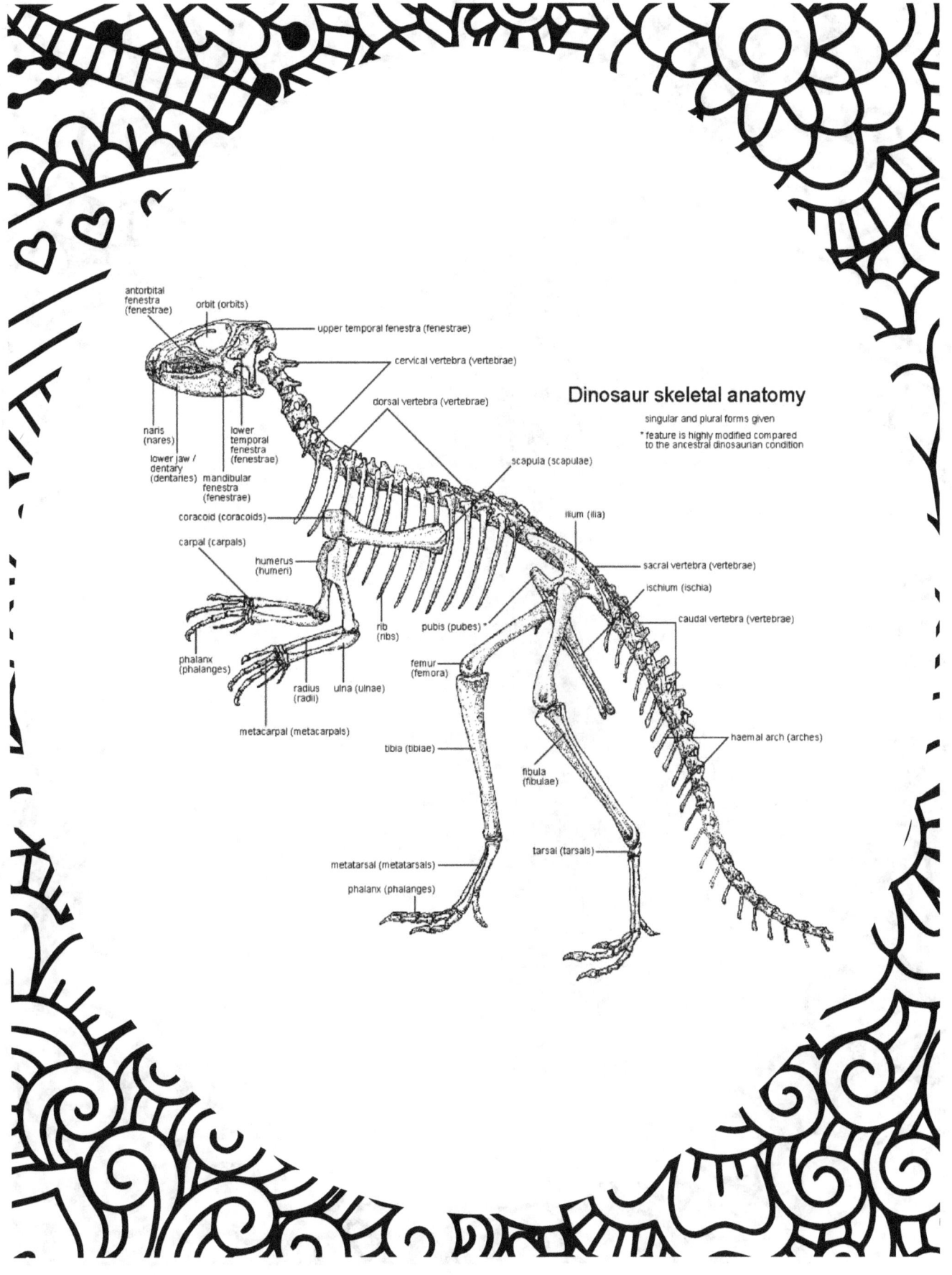

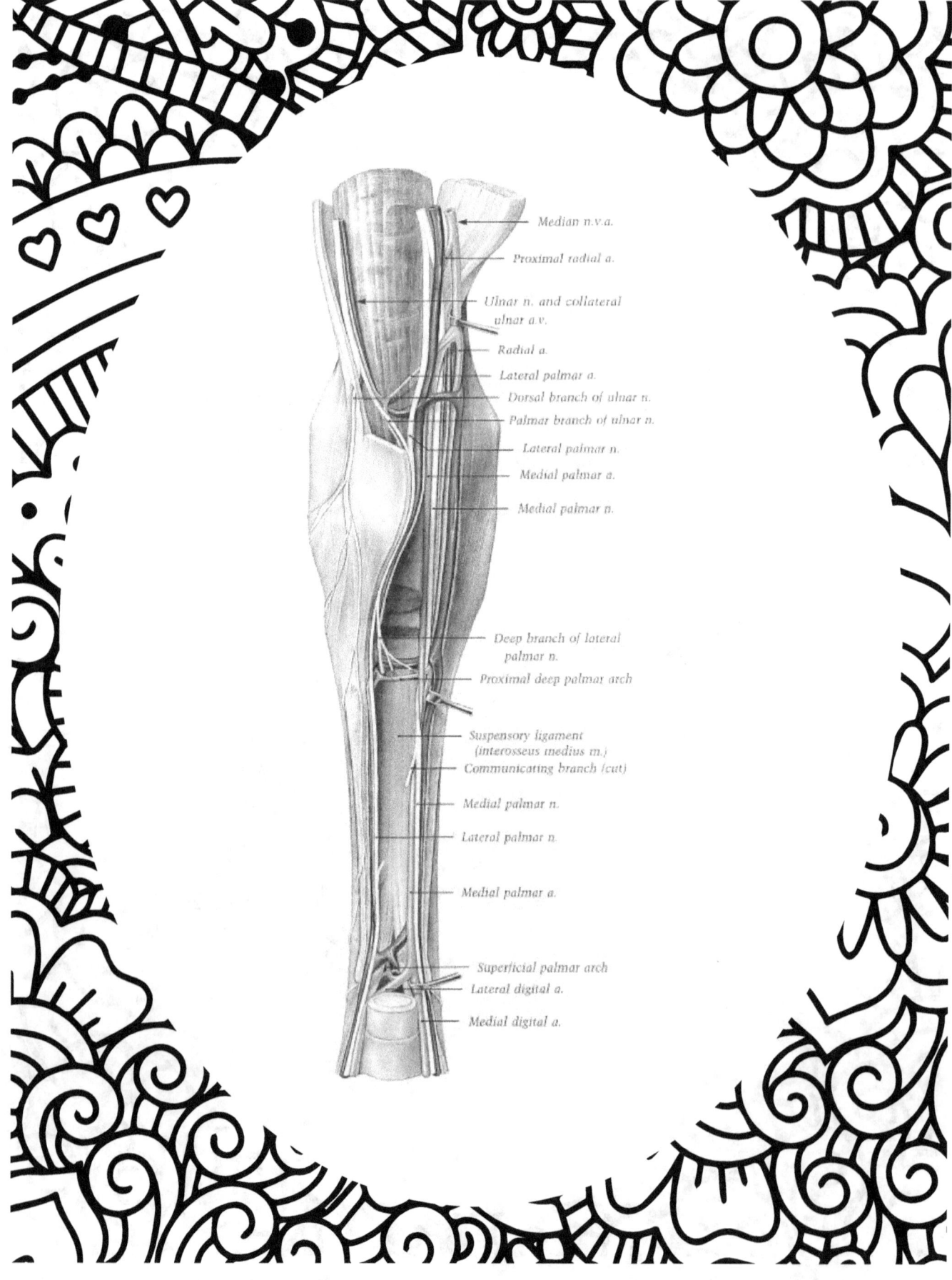

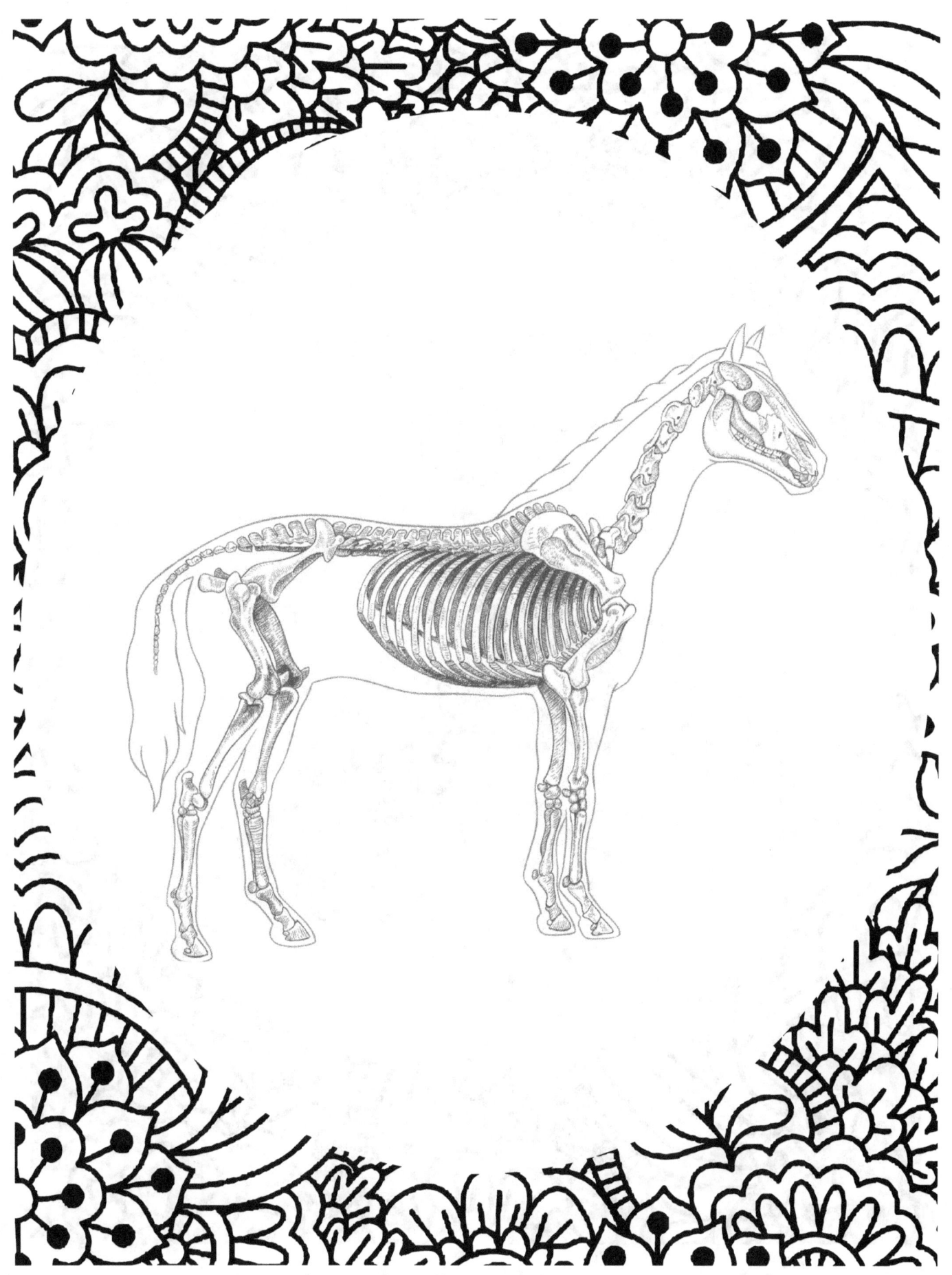

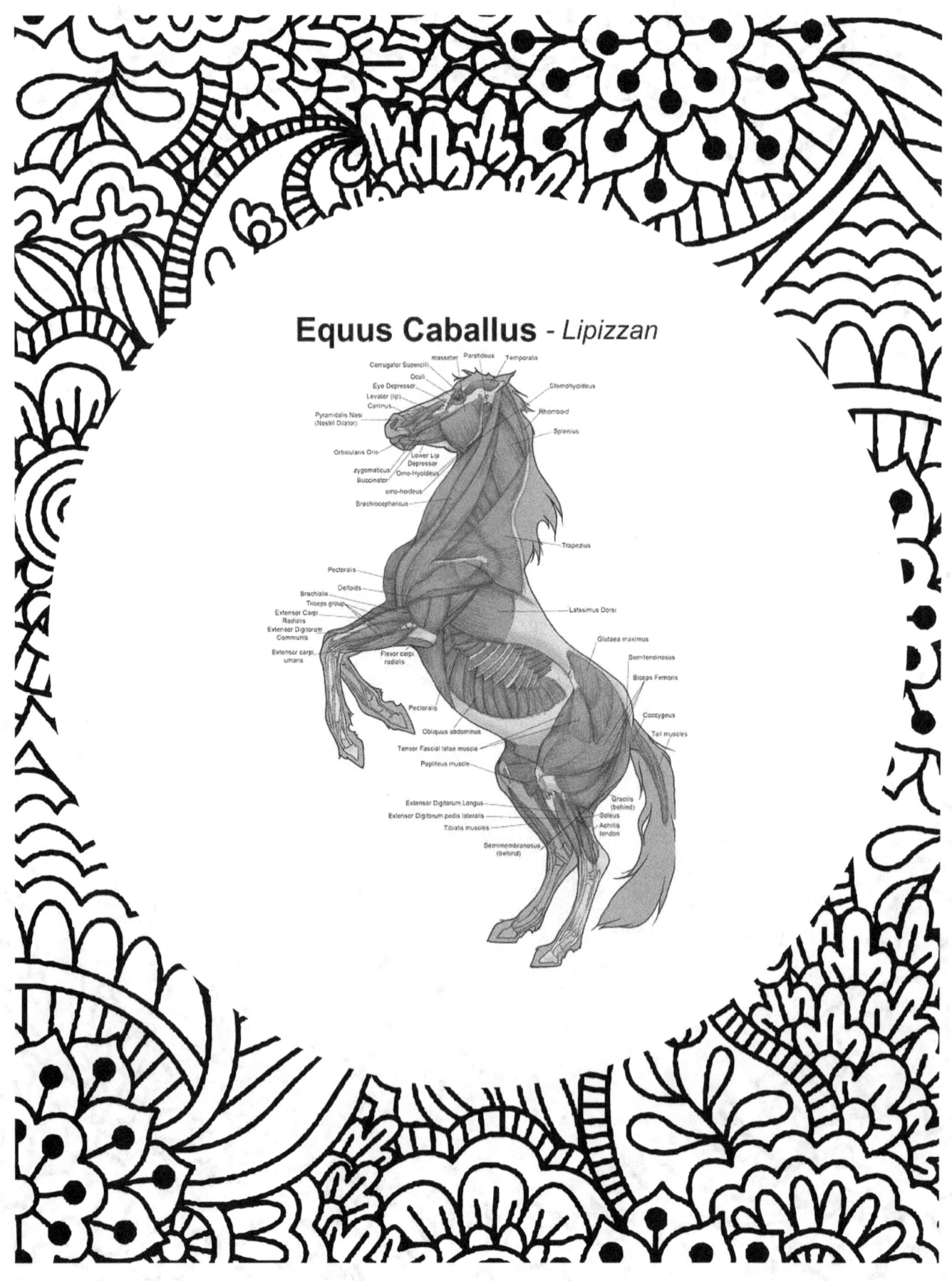

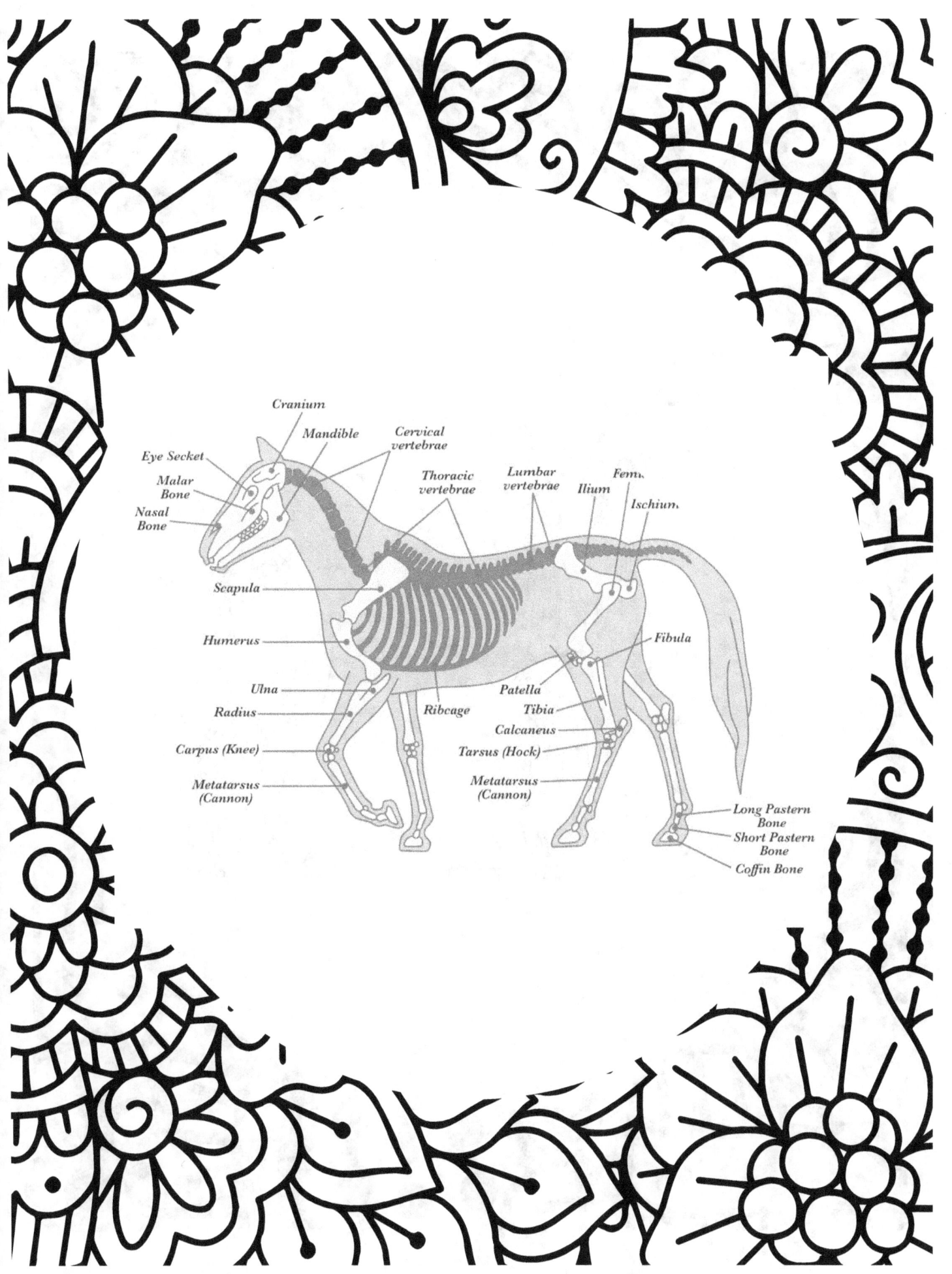

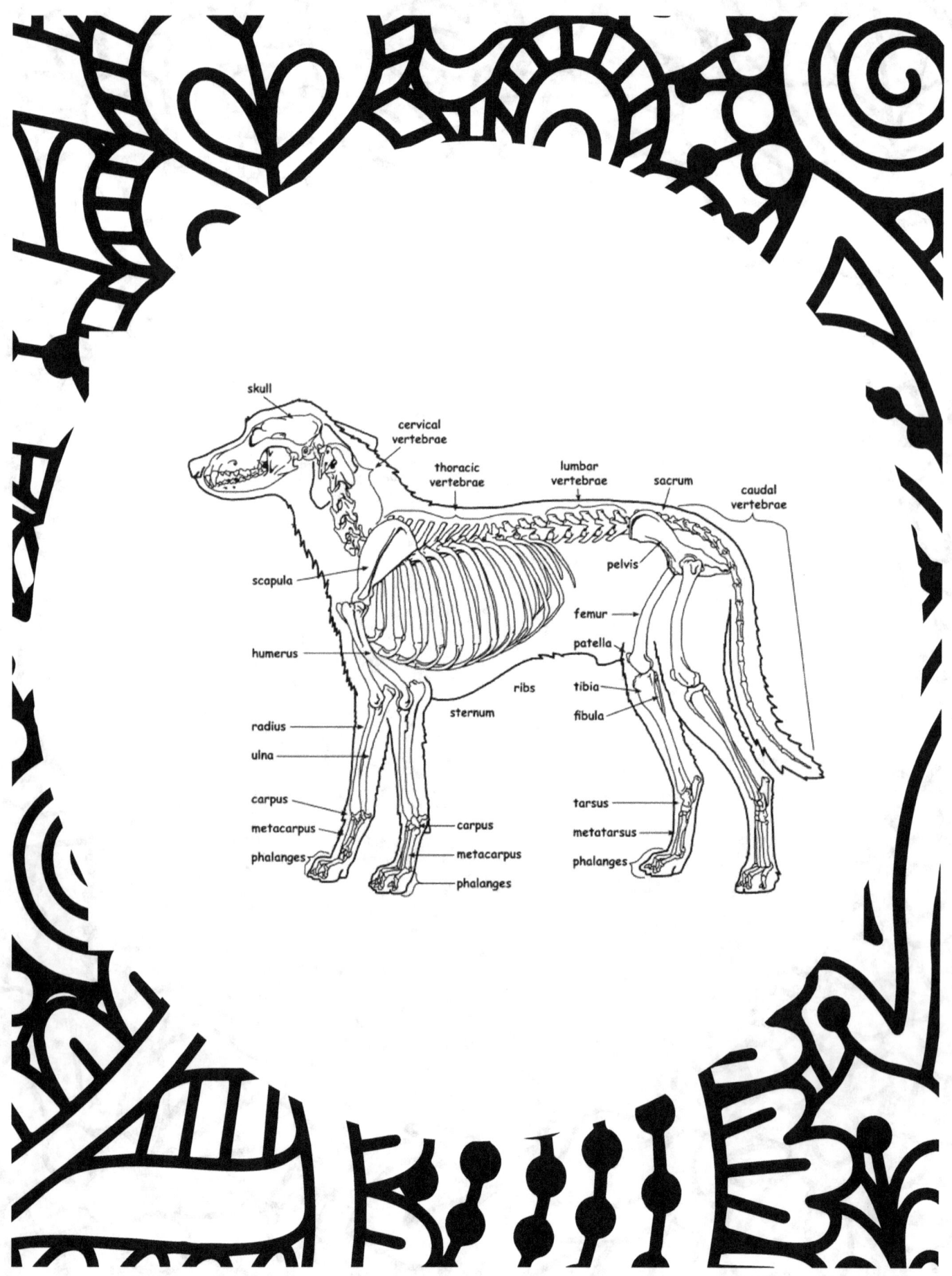

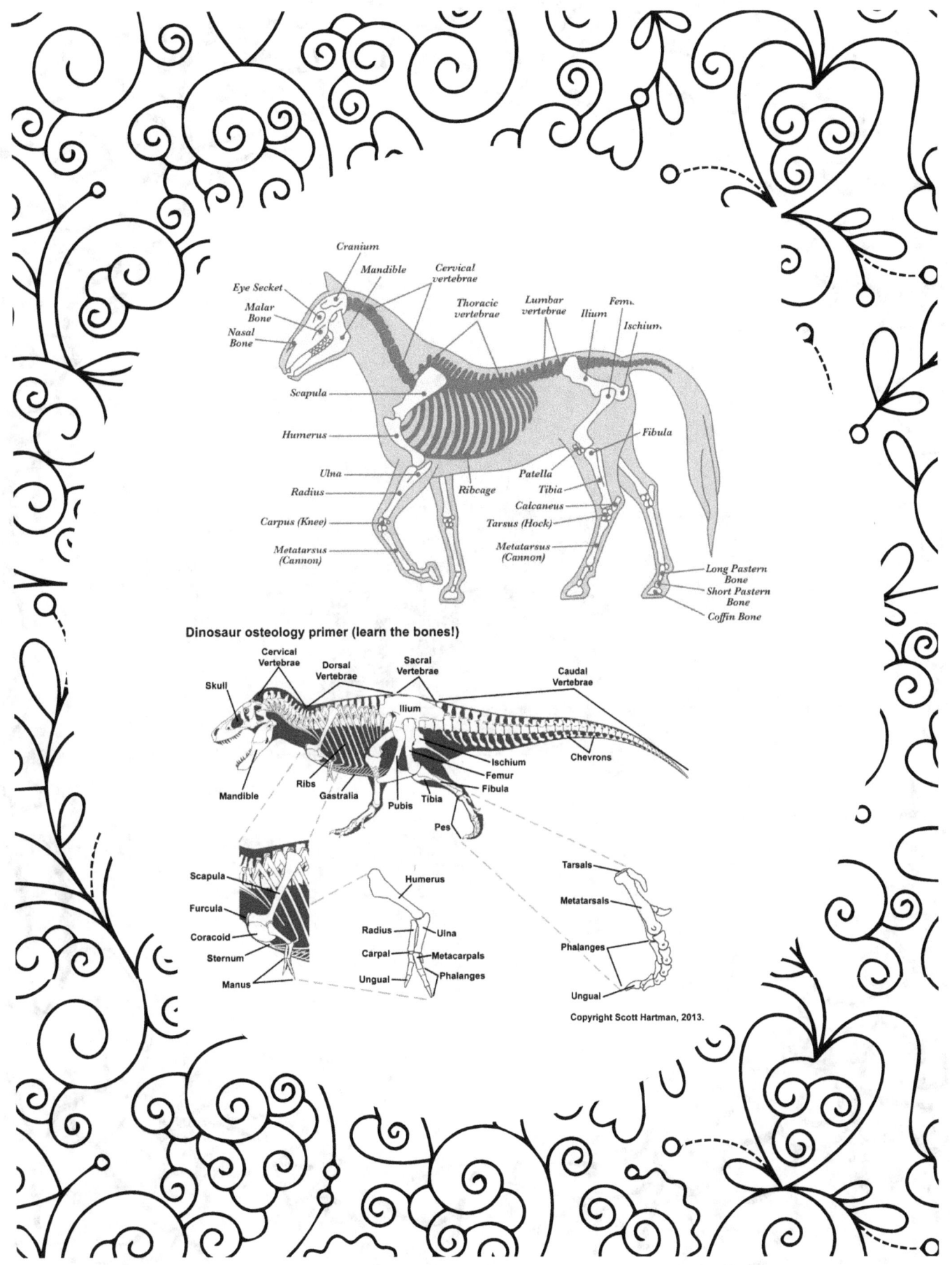

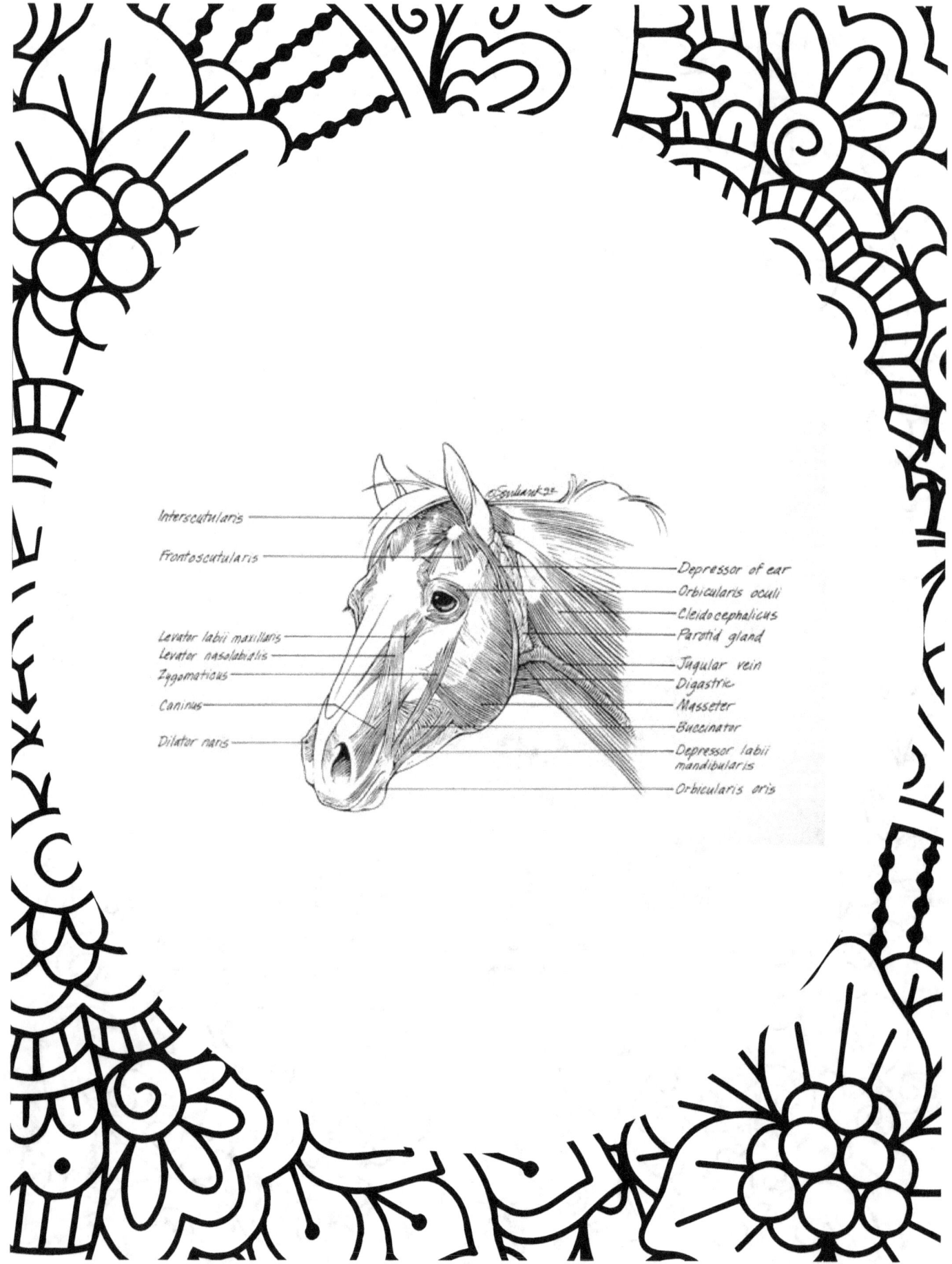

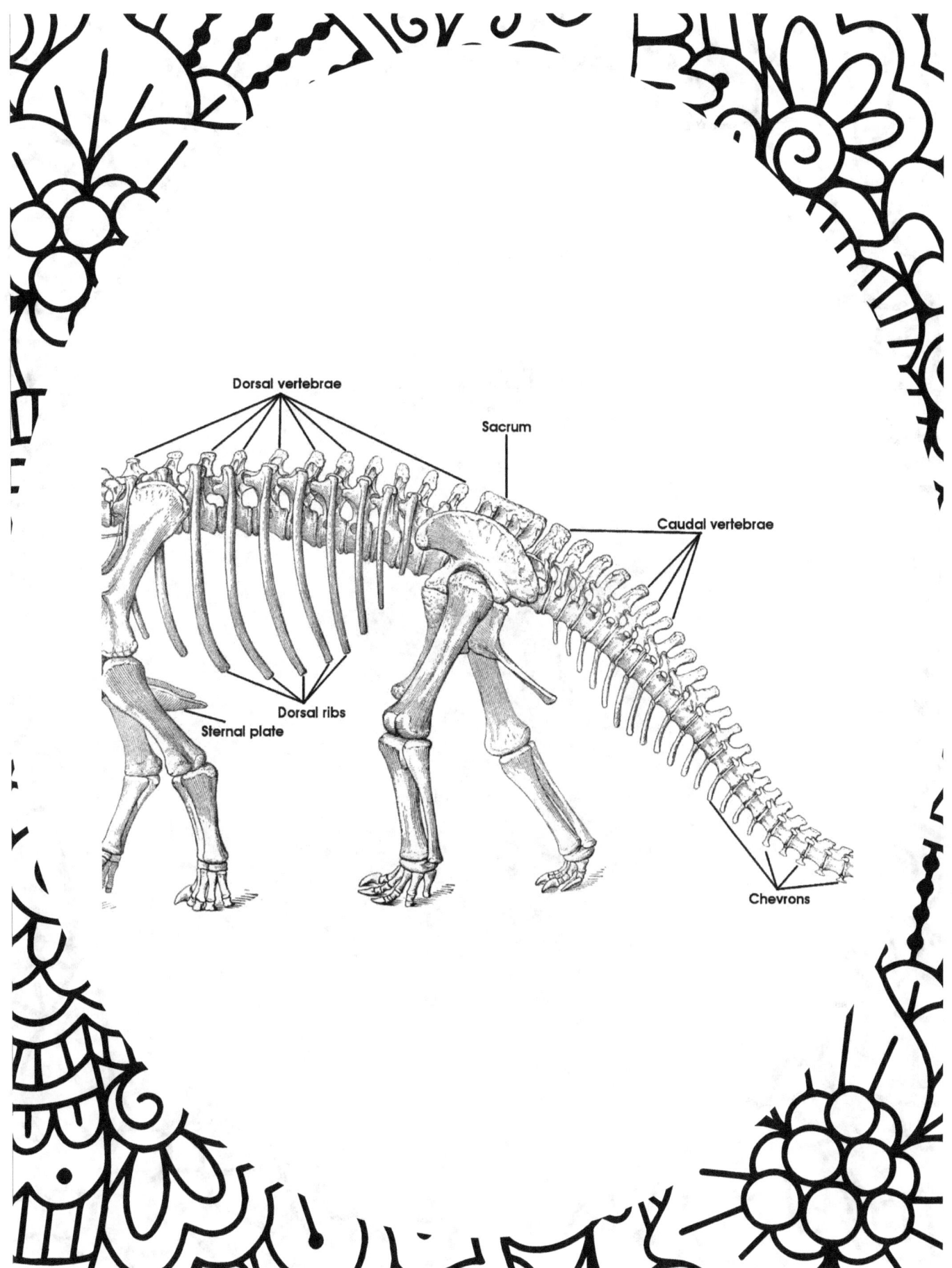

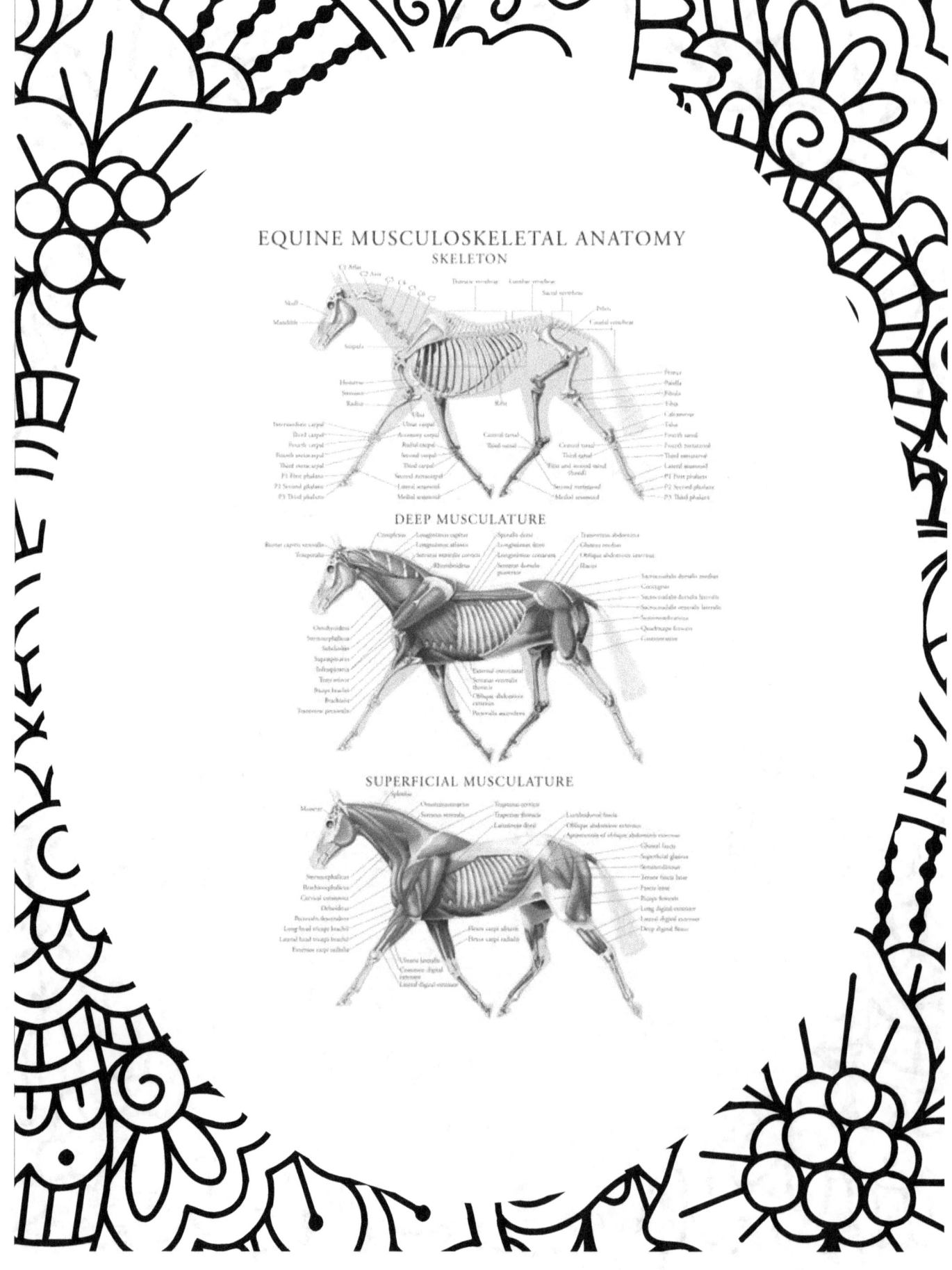

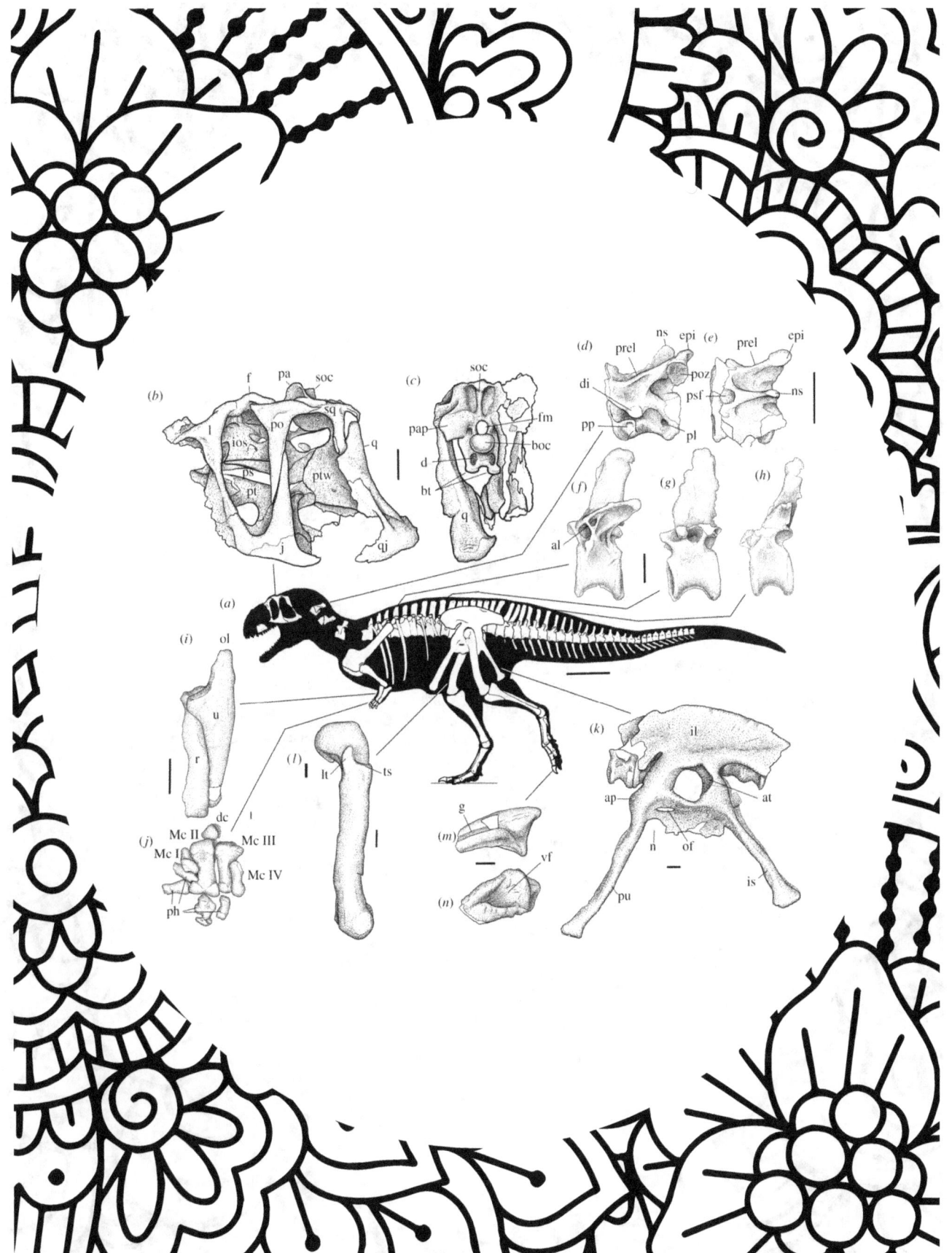

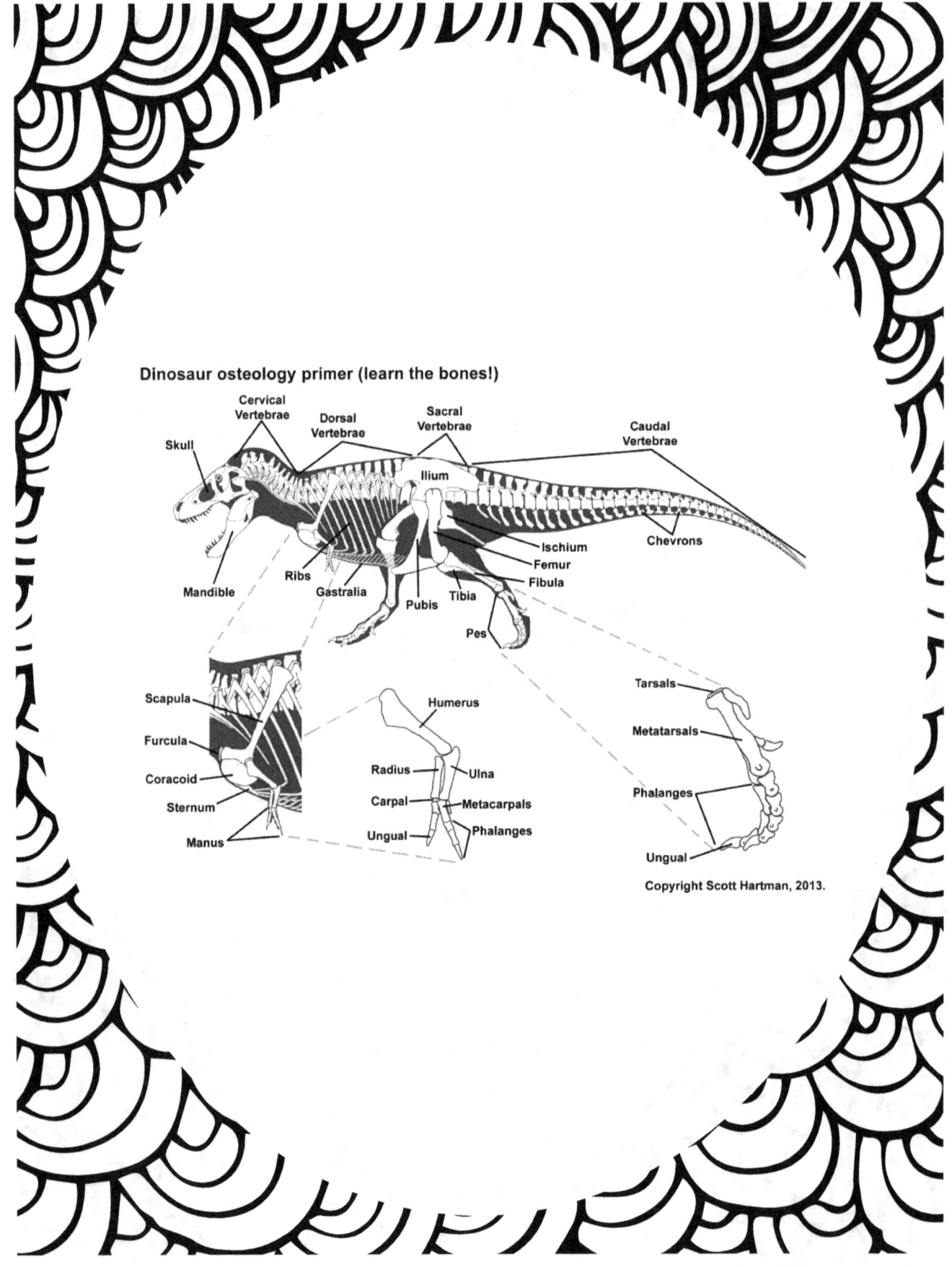

www.ingramcontent.com/pod-product-compliance
Lightning Source LLC
Chambersburg PA
CBHW081701220526
45466CB00009B/2847